Evidence-based Practice in Nursing

Transforming Nursing Practice series

Transforming Nursing Practice is the first series of books designed to help students meet the requirements of the NMC Standards and Essential Skills Clusters for degree programmes. Each book addresses a core topic, and together they cover the generic knowledge required for all fields of practice. Accessible and challenging, *Transforming Nursing Practice* helps nursing students prepare for the demands of future healthcare delivery.

Core knowledge titles:

Series editor: Dr Shirley Bach, Head of the School of Nursing and Midwifery at the University of Brighton

Communication and Interpersonal Skills in Nursing (2nd. ed)	ISBN 978 0 85725 449 8
Contexts of Contemporary Nursing (2nd. ed.)	ISBN 978 1 84445 374 0
Health Promotion and Public Health in Nursing	ISBN 978 0 85725 437 5
Introduction to Medicines Management in Nursing	ISBN 978 1 84445 845 5
Law and Professional Issues in Nursing (2nd. ed.)	ISBN 978 1 84445 372 6
Leadership, Management and Team Working in Nursing	ISBN 978 0 85725 453 5
Learning Skills for Nursing Students	ISBN 978 1 84445 376 4
Medicines Management in Adult Nursing	ISBN 978 1 84445 842 4
Medicines Management in Children's Nursing	ISBN 978 1 84445 470 9
Medicines Management in Mental Health Nursing	ISBN 978 0 85725 049 0
Nursing Adults with Long Term Conditions	ISBN 978 0 85725 441 2
Nursing and Collaborative Practice (2nd. ed)	ISBN 978 1 84445 373 3
Nursing and Mental Health Care	ISBN 978 1 84445 467 9
Passing Calculations Tests for Nursing Students	ISBN 978 1 84445 471 6
Patient and Carer Participation in Nursing	ISBN 978 0 85725 307 1
Successful Practice Learning for Nursing Students (2nd. ed)	ISBN 978 0 85725 315 6
What is Nursing? Exploring Theory and Practice (2nd. ed.)	ISBN 978 0 85725 445 0

Personal and professional learning skills titles:

Series editors: Dr Mooi Standing, Independent Academic Consultant at national and international level and Dr Shirley Bach, Head of the School of Nursing and Midwifery at the University of Brighton

Clinical Judgement and Decision Making in Nursing	ISBN 978 1 84445 468 6
Critical Thinking and Writing for Nursing Students	ISBN 978 1 84445 366 5
Evidence-based Practice in Nursing	ISBN 978 1 84445 369 6
Information Skills for Nursing Students	ISBN 978 1 84445 381 8
Reflective Practice in Nursing	ISBN 978 1 84445 371 9
Succeeding in Research Project Plans and Literature Reviews for Nursing Students	ISBN 978 0 85725 264 7
Successful Professional Portfolios for Nursing Students	ISBN 978 0 85725 457 3
Understanding Research for Nursing Students	ISBN 978 1 84445 368 9

You can also find more information on each of these titles and our other learning resources at www.learningmatters.co.uk. Many of these titles are also available in various e-book formats, please visit our website for more information.

Evidence-based Practice in Nursing

Peter Ellis

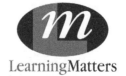

LearningMatters

First published in 2010 by Learning Matters Ltd
Reprinted twice in 2011

British Library Cataloguing in Publication Data
A CIP record for this book is available from the British Library

ISBN: 978 1 84445 369 6

This book is also available in the following ebook formats:

Adobe ebook   ISBN: 978 1 84445 749 6
EPUB ebook   ISBN: 978 1 84445 748 9
Kindle   ISBN: 978 0 85725 015 5

Cover design by Toucan Design
Project Management by Diana Chambers
Typeset by Kelly Winter
Printed and bound in Great Britain by MPG Books Group

Learning Matters Ltd
20 Cathedral Yard
Exeter EX1 1HB
Tel: 01392 215560
E-mail: info@learningmatters.co.uk
www.learningmatters.co.uk

Contents

Foreword

This is an excellent book that captures and portrays the complexity of evidence-based practice in nursing in a refreshingly thoughtful, imaginative, informative and practical way. It is very rare for nurses to be able to pick up a book and think 'Yes, I can totally relate to that' or 'It says everything about nursing I know to be true but have not been able to say myself' or 'At last, a book about evidence-based practice that actually validates nurses' knowledge, skills and experience in addition to formal research evidence'. This is such a book!

Peter Ellis has succeeded, where many others have only aspired, in 'putting his finger' on an elusive truth about a continually changing broad spectrum of information sources influencing everyday clinical practice in providing high-quality patient-centred care. This 'kaleidoscopic' effect of multiple interweaving types of evidence is creatively and skilfully presented in an innovative model of the influences on and dispositions of an evidence-based nurse. It identifies various types of evidence including research, practical knowledge/experience, health policy, patient preferences, legal or ethical issues, and inter-professional feedback, and shows how each of these are evaluated, applied and combined to inform patient-centred care.

In order to appreciate and harness the important contribution each type of evidence makes to patient-centred care (and be able to access, review and apply them) Peter identifies a range of 'dispositions of the evidence-based nurse' that we need to cultivate as nurses, including being a questioning, critical and creative thinker, reflective and reflexive, morally active, self-aware and considerate of others. This is invaluable in showing us that the qualities we associate with our professional identity as nurses, and take pride in, are valued. This is vital for helping us to ensure that the best available evidence is applied for the benefit of our patients.

The reader is carefully guided and challenged to develop and apply the attributes needed to understand how different types of evidence can enhance patient care throughout the book. Thankfully, it is more a case of 'do as I do' as opposed to 'do as I say (but cannot do myself)' and readers will appreciate how the realities of practice are clearly related to the theory and research presented in the book. I am very pleased to have been able make a small contribution to this important book, and I highly recommend it.

Dr Mooi Standing
Series Editor

About the authors

Peter Ellis is Senior Lecturer in Nursing and Applied Clinical Studies at Canterbury Christ Church University, where he teaches on research modules from foundation degree to Masters level. Peter is a specialist renal nurse with higher degrees in Health Care Ethics and Medical Epidemiology. Prior to joining Canterbury Christ Church University, Peter was Senior Nurse – Renal Outpatients and Research Projects Manager at King's College Hospital, London.

Contributors

Lioba Howatson-Jones is Senior Lecturer in the Department of Nursing and Applied Clinical Studies at Canterbury Christ Church University. Lioba teaches on a variety of modules from undergraduate to Masters level and is particularly interested in academic development reflecting her doctoral research in Education. Her background is in surgical and ambulatory care, and in practice development.

Kay Hutchfield began her nursing career in both orthopaedic nursing and adult nursing before becoming a children's nurse and later a clinical teacher. She has recently retired after 18 years as a senior lecturer in higher education. She has worked primarily in pre-registration nursing education, and has a keen interest in curriculum development. Kay has been programme director for three pre-registration child nursing programmes, and has developed a keen interest in developing students' fundamental research skills and managing risk in academic work as well as in care management. Kay has a particular interest in information literacy and graduate skills development.

Dr Mooi Standing is an Independent Academic Consultant. Mooi provides consultancy in international partnership development, curriculum planning, quality enhancement and continuing professional development both nationally and internationally. Mooi practiced mental health and general nursing in various hospital and community settings and has over 20 years experience in nursing training/ education working within a higher education institution environment. Mooi is actively involved in the development of collaborative nursing and health care programmes at undergraduate and post graduate levels internationally. She has contributed to a number of undergraduate nursing books and has published papers in various peer reviewed journals on the subject of clinical decision-making and hermeneutic phenomenology. Mooi is also an accredited Nursing and Midwifery Council (NMC) reviewer, approving, monitoring and assuring the quality of nursing programmes throughout the United Kingdom.

Introduction

One of the enduring tensions of nursing is the theory–practice gap. Some practising nurses regard this as an inevitable consequence of the move towards degree-level nursing in the UK where academics are seen as being far removed from the realities of practice while some academics regard this as being a result of practising nurses' hesitance to engage in degree-level education.

Whatever the reality of the theory–practice gap, the conscientious adoption of a coherent framework for the progression of practice through engagement with personal development and new sources of information, while maintaining a view on the realities of clinical nursing, might well help solve this dilemma.

In this book we take the view that the purpose of academic nursing is to support the enhancement of practice. To achieve this it is necessary that academic nursing takes account of the nature and realities of clinical practice. To this end we present a view of evidence-based practice that is both grounded in academic nursing (information, knowledge, evidence) and practical nursing (experience, reflection, reflexivity and patient preference). What seems clear to us in presenting this argument is that nursing is a practical undertaking and we cannot and should not engage in the creation of evidence that does not support this.

The subsequent sections will enable you to gain an overview of the messages contained within the book and how these might fit together to inform your development as an action-oriented evidence-driven nurse.

Chapter 1, Towards an inclusive model of evidence-based care: this introductory chapter sets the scene for the rest of the book and demonstrates how the various strands of evidence might be drawn together to create an inclusive picture of evidence-based nursing practice. It also examines some of the dispositions and characteristics that it might be necessary for a nurse to adopt in order to become truly evidence-based.

Chapter 2, Sources of knowledge for evidence-based care: access to information is easier now than it has ever been. The internet provides the nurse with access to sources of information that are both immediate and accessible. Newspapers, television, journals and other media carry stories about issues that affect not only health but the ways in which healthcare is delivered. The novice nurse may be tempted to use these sources of information in an unquestioning way, readily accepting what they say as being applicable to nursing practice. The more experienced nurse, or student, may feel that other sources of information are more appropriate, for instance nursing journals and professional internet-based nursing resources.

While more faith can be placed in professional sources of information, we argue in this book that there remains a need to show some caution in the sourcing and interpretation of sources of knowledge, and that even the best sources of information for practice require that the evidence-based nurse applies some criteria to judging the truth and usefulness of the information these sources contain.

Chapter 3, *Critiquing research: the generic elements*: any book about evidence-based practice (EBP) cannot ignore the contribution of research to the nursing evidence base. Unlike many other books about EBP, this book regards research as being of only equal importance as other sources of knowledge. Chapter 3 will explore methods for critiquing the elements of research that appear in all research papers.

Chapter 4, *Critiquing research: approach-specific elements*: this is a continuation of Chapter 3 and seeks to expand upon the critiquing of research that is undertaken in either the qualitative or quantitative paradigm. The appendix to this chapter, which is a critiquing framework, should be read alongside Chapters 3 and 4, as together they are intended to provide guidance of the critiquing of research for either academic purposes or to inform practice.

Chapter 5, *Making sense of subjective experience*: a fundamental aspect of being able to draw on many sources of information at once and to make sense of what one is hearing and seeing is having the ability to be both reflective and reflexive. Rather than explain how these strategies are practised (which is explored in the book *Reflective practice in nursing* in this series), Chapter 5 examines how they can contribute to our understanding of sources of evidence other than research, namely subjective knowledge.

Chapter 6, *Working with others*: here we explore collaborative working as a strategy for improving our evidence base for practice. The chapter explores how we as nurses can use others to develop ourselves and our understanding of care delivery. Working with others means working with different health and social care professionals (which is explored in the book *Nursing and collaborative practice*, also in this series) and, most importantly, patients themselves. Evidence-based practice requires nurses to be aware of, respond to and engage with the input of all individuals involved with an episode of care.

Chapter 7, *Clinical decision making in evidence-based practice*: this chapter considers how the nurse might draw together various sources of evidence, reconcile the various influences on practice and apply the skills identified in earlier chapters in order to make worthwhile clinical decisions with individual patients. It challenges the reader to think about the ethical context of their decisions and how these affect individual patients, and draws together the threads of the arguments presented in the other chapters and creates a practical guide to clinical decision making. (The issues identified in this chapter are explored in more depth in *Clinical judgement and decision-making for nursing students*, also in this series.)

Chapter 8: *Getting evidence into practice*: here we explore some mechanisms by which evidence may be translated into meaningful practice. This chapter examines the social, practical and human barriers to the use of evidence in practice. It examines barriers to change and how change management strategies might be used to overcome these. It concentrates on personal and team strategies to support the adoption of evidence and what benefits might accrue from these.

NMC *Standards for pre-registration nursing education* and Essential Skills Clusters

The Nursing and Midwifery Council (NMC) has standards of competence that have to be met by applicants to different parts of the nursing and midwifery register. These standards are what they deem as being necessary for the delivery of safe, effective nursing and midwifery practice.

As well as specific competencies, the NMC identifies specific skills nursing students must have at various points of their training programme. These Essential Skills Clusters (ESCs) are essential abilities that students need to attain in order to practise to their full potential.

This book includes the latest standards for 2010 onwards, taken from *Standards for Pre-registration Nursing Education* (NMC, 2010). For links to the pre-2010 standards, please visit the website for the book at **www.learningmatters.co.uk/nursing**.

Activities

At various stages within each chapter there are points at which you can break to undertake various activities. Undertaking and understanding the activities is an important and integral element of your understanding of the content of each chapter. You are encouraged, where appropriate, to reflect on your practice and how the things you have learned from working with patients might inform your understanding of research. Other activities will require that you take time away from the book to find out new information that will add to your understanding of the topic under discussion. Some activities challenge you to apply your learning to a question or scenario to help you think about a theme in more depth in order to add to your understanding. A few activities require that you make observations during your day-to-day life or in the clinical setting. These activities are designed to increase your understanding of the topics under discussion and how they reflect on nursing practice.

Where appropriate, there are suggested or potential answers to activities at the end of the chapter. It is recommended that you try, where possible, to engage with the activities in order to increase your understanding of the realities of nursing research.

Words that are in **bold** in the chapters relate to words that are included in the glossary that has been added to aid your reading of the book.

We hope you find the book both informative and enjoyable.

Chapter 1

Towards an inclusive model of evidence-based care

Peter Ellis

Chapter aims

After reading this chapter, you will be able to:

- understand that evidence for practice comes in many forms;
- identify key components of the evidence base for practice;
- understand why evidence for practice is important;
- begin to create a coherent picture of what critical practice actually means.

Introduction

Nurses work in ever changing environments of care. Changes in governmental and local policy, improvements in technology and pharmaceuticals, the changing demography of the world and developments in society all impact on the ways in which we deliver care to our patients. Not only do we face the challenge of a constantly changing and evolving workplace, but as a student nurse you have to try to make sense of what you learn in the classroom and how this relates to the realities of what you experience in the workplace. As a staff nurse the pressures increase somewhat as you continue to work in an ever changing environment, one that requires that you evolve and develop with it in order to deliver high-quality care, for which you are now professionally accountable.

All of the pressures of care delivery can lead to an overwhelming feeling of helplessness. Perhaps you feel that you might not know all that you think you should know before you go onto the wards, or that what you have learnt might well be out of date soon. Being prepared for life as a nurse requires you to embrace the many opportunities for lifelong learning so you can develop skills in identifying and evaluating information (evidence) that will stand you in good stead throughout your nursing career.

This chapter seeks to set the scene for the rest of the book in describing an attitude and approach to learning and development that will help support you, as a student or trained nurse, in making sense of where you work and what you do in practice. It is the aim of this chapter to stimulate you to think about how and why you practise in the way you do and how you can make sense of the various influences on your practice.

This approach might seem at odds with an evidence-based practice approach to care; after all, isn't evidence all about being able to access, critique and apply research to practice? In this book we take the view that research is not the only source of knowledge for practice – nor should it be. We take the view, and present the argument, that in order to truly act in an evidential way in practice, the nurse needs to knit together many sources of evidence. The position we take is that sources of knowledge may stand alone as evidence or may serve to validate or refute other sources of evidence. For example, a randomised controlled trial may demonstrate the worth of a 'keep fit' intervention for weight loss, and this evidence may be validated by a qualitative enquiry that shows that the people involved enjoy the keep fit and want to do it. Conversely, they may not enjoy the process and therefore the intervention will ultimately fail.

In this book we demonstrate that all the different sources of information and influences on the way in which nursing is practised are potentially of equal importance at one time or another. We further show that to nurse effectively in the twenty-first century, and beyond, requires you to be able to identify and use all forms of information in order to turn them into evidence that will be used to inform practice.

In order to achieve this, this chapter explores some of the influences that have shaped nursing practice. It describes and explores the rise of evidence-based practice and develops a big-picture view of how you can prepare yourself for the challenges of modern practice. Rising to this challenge requires you to adopt a constantly questioning approach to your practice that is both beneficial to your learning and working life, and, ultimately and importantly, to your patients.

Activity 1.1   *Reflection*

Try to remember what made you want to study to become a nurse in the first place. Stop and think about what you thought would inform and guide what you would do in your everyday practice as a nurse before you became a nursing student. Talk to others on your programme about what they felt or thought about this.

As this is based on your own reflection there is no answer for this activity at the end of the chapter.

Why evidence-based nursing is important

There is a culture of increasing scrutiny of the work of health and social care professionals which has come about, at least in part, in response to various scandals (see the case studies in the box below). Such very public scandals have contributed to a climate of care in which nurses are increasingly required to be able to justify the decisions they make with and for patients. No longer is it good enough for nurses to claim they know what is best for their patients just because they are nurses. The rise in patient power and the governmental agenda of service user consultation and involvement (DH, 1989, 1991, 2001) have created a climate of care in which nurses have to be able to justify not only what they do but also how and why they are doing it.

CASE STUDY: *Some of the scandals that have affected healthcare in the UK*

On 25 February 2000, Victoria Climbié died after years of neglect and abuse from her aunt and her boyfriend. In his report of the inquiry into the death of Victoria, Lord Laming states: *I found it hard to understand why established good medical practice, that would have undoubtedly helped clarify the complexities in Victoria's case, was not followed.*

In January 2001 the Redfern report criticised the actions of a pathologist at the children's hospital, Alder Hey, for removing and retaining human organs and tissue samples without consent. The public outcry that followed led the UK government to publish new guidelines outlining the law on the handling of human body parts (**www.rlcinquiry.org.uk**).

On 15 April 2009 Margaret Haywood was struck off the Nursing and Midwifery Council's register for secretly filming the alleged neglect of elderly patients at the Royal Sussex Hospital. The public response to the programme had been one of outrage.

There is no doubting that nursing takes place very much in the public eye, and when nurses and other health and social care professionals make mistakes, they come in for severe criticism. There is also without a doubt a feeling in society at large that all care professionals should know what they are doing, why they are doing it and do it well.

Such expectations are daunting but very understandable, and most nurses aspire to live up to these very reasonable expectations. Clearly, knowledge of what evidence-based practice is will not be sufficient for you to meet these expectations; however, knowledge of how you might go about identifying evidence to inform practice and how you might subsequently assimilate this evidence into your practice will be. In short, evidence-based nursing practice is not a purely academic exercise; it is a means of knitting together knowledge from a number of different sources in a way that has the potential to impact positively on what we do as nurses: care.

Activity 1.2   Reflection

Think about a time that you, or a family member, were a patient. How well do you feel you were kept informed about the care you received and why it was being delivered in the way it was? Ask a more experienced colleague what is was like to be a nurse in the past and how the evidence-based care agenda has changed the way in which care is delivered. Do they think it is a good thing or a bad thing? Why?

There are some possible answers and thoughts at the end of the chapter.

Knowing what you are doing and why informs part of an important element of modern nursing and healthcare practice called **clinical governance**. Clinical governance is a system whereby what nurses, and other care professionals, do in practice is subjected to scrutiny to ensure it is worthwhile and money is being spent wisely. The National Institute for Health and Clinical Excellence (NICE) and National Service Frameworks (NSFs) create guidelines and policies about how NHS money is used. They use evidence from many sources to inform the policies that they produce, and these are widely regarded as guides to good practice.

Activity 1.3   Research and finding out

Have a look at an NSF or some NICE guidelines on a subject you know something about. Pay particular attention to what evidence informed the decision making and who was involved in drawing up the guidance.

The website addresses for NICE and some key NSFs are given at the end of the chapter in the Useful websites section.

Not only is the requirement to evidence what we do as nurses a result of political and social pressure, but there are good moral reasons as to why nurses need to show that what they are doing is in the best interests of their patients. Accountability is a central tenet of the Nursing and Midwifery Council's *Code* of conduct, performance and ethics (2008), which states that: *As a professional, you are personally accountable for actions and omissions in your practice and must always be able to justify your decisions.*

Beauchamp and Childress (2007) argue that ethical practice in healthcare requires that the providers of care, including nurses and student nurses, are mindful of what they term the four principles of healthcare ethics. These are:

- beneficence (doing good);
- non-maleficence (avoiding unnecessary harm);

- autonomy (respecting freedom of action);
- justice (fairness).

Activity 1.4   *Critical thinking*

There are, of course, a number of other ethical approaches that might inform how we act as nurses, but the message from Beauchamp and Childress has clear connections as to why evidence is important in nursing. Stop for a while and think about what these might be. Perhaps you might like to look for some further definitions of the four principles and think about why they are important in establishing the importance of evidence-based care.

Some ideas as to how these might apply and references to sources for further definitions of the principles are given at the end of the chapter.

In the UK, we are used to idea that healthcare is provided 'free at the point of use'; indeed, this is one of the founding principles of the National Health Service, and one of the things that makes it such a special institution in which people hold great pride. However, 'free at the point of use' is not the same as 'free'. The money that funds the activity of the NHS comes directly out of the public purse; it is money that is raised through taxation and national insurance contributions and, as such, it is money that needs to be spent wisely. There are many pressures on how NHS money is used, and to spend money on futile practices means that there is less money available elsewhere in the system for other things. The use of evidence in practice is therefore essential in order to help make the money available go as far as it can reasonably be expected to. The idea of getting good value for money links strongly to the concepts of ethics and governance discussed above.

Recent developments in nursing and in healthcare in general – for example, the increase in advanced practitioner and nurse consultant roles as well as the move from hospital to community-based care – have had a dramatic impact on the ways in which nurses practise. The need for an increase in autonomous working while supporting and developing interprofessional and patient-centred approaches to care means that the nurse is required to *use evidence-based knowledge from nursing and related disciplines to select and individualise nursing interventions* (NMC, 2004). Such decision making requires that the nurse is familiar with the most current evidence and how this applies to the situations that arise in their practice.

Traditionally, nursing practice was built on an apprenticeship model whereby the student learnt to nurse in a manner that reflected what was deemed to represent good nursing by the ward sister and the staff nurses on the ward. As such, the way in which nursing care was delivered was based on historical ways of working that had been passed down between generations of nurses with little change and little in the way of questioning. Such practices can become ritualised and are practised because that is what we have always done. Not all nursing traditions are bad or detrimental; for example, the regular changing of linen and bedding – at one time more a matter of pleasing matron than anything else – is now known to play a role in infection control. However, some traditions are at odds with the notions of evidence-based practice that are presented in this book primarily because they are undertaken in an unquestioning and unthinking way.

In this section we have identified that there are a number of reasons why evidence-based practice for nursing is essential. We have seen that adopting evidence-informed ways of working is not an optional extra that nurses can ignore if they are too busy. Key among the reasons for adopting a questioning and evidence-based approach to care provision are the ethical arguments about doing good and avoiding harm, the wise use of resources and the development of nursing as a more autonomous profession. In the next section we will examine what evidence-based practice might actually mean.

Definitions of evidence-based practice

There has been – and there remains – some debate about what evidence-based practice actually means. There are many definitions of evidence-based practice, research-informed practice, evidence-based medicine, evidence-based healthcare and evidence-based nursing in the literature. Before we go on to define what we mean by evidence-based practice in this book, and before we explore the concepts that might inform such practice for nursing, it is worth exploring some of these definitions in an attempt to get a feel for what EBP might actually be.

The number and diversity of the definitions demonstrate that there is little agreement between professionals within healthcare as to what exactly evidence-based care means. This can be a source of confusion for the student nurse, who should take time to reflect upon what they thought nursing practice was based on before they started nursing, once they started nursing and again as they become more familiar with nursing practice.

Polit and Beck (2008, p3) define evidence-based practice as:

the use of best clinical evidence in making patient care decisions ... such evidence typically comes from research conducted by nurses and other health care professionals.

This definition places research squarely at the centre of clinical decision making and recognises that such research may come from sources other than just the nursing profession.

Perhaps the most widely quoted definition comes from Sackett et al. (1996, p71), who defined evidence-based medicine as:

the conscientious, explicit and judicious use of current best evidence in making decisions about the care of the individual patient. It means integrating individual clinical expertise with the best available external clinical evidence from systematic research.

This definition identifies a number of important markers of evidence-based practice.

- It is conscientious – it is a purposeful activity that one chooses to engage in.
- It is explicit – it is applied in such a way that it can be shown to have been used.

- It is judicious – thought has been given to how it applies to the job in hand.
- It is about the care of the individual patient – the evidence fits the situation one is dealing with.
- It is a mix of individual expertise with knowledge that has been gathered from good quality research.

What Sackett et al. are saying is that one answer will not fit all clinical scenarios and that it is the role of the doctor, in this case, to identify the research that best fits the clinical situation that is in front of them. McKibbon (1998, p399) provides a more far-reaching and inclusive definition.

> *Evidence-based practice (EBP) is an approach to health care wherein health professionals use the best evidence possible, i.e. the most appropriate information available, to make clinical decisions for individual patients. EBP values, enhances and builds on clinical expertise, knowledge of disease mechanisms, and pathophysiology. It involves complex and conscientious decision-making based not only on the available evidence but also on patient characteristics, situations, and preferences. It recognizes that health care is individualized and ever changing and involves uncertainties and probabilities. Ultimately EBP is the formalization of the care process that the best clinicians have practiced for generations.*

This explanation of EBP goes beyond the other two definitions in recognising the importance of the patient in making decisions ('preferences') about their own care and, as such, perhaps better reflects modern nursing practice as we see it.

If we are to move the concept of EBP in nursing forward, it is perhaps best to attach it to well-established, patient-focused strategies with which nurses are all familiar. The nursing process of assessing, planning, implementing and evaluating care can be seen to be similar to the stages of implementing EBP that Hek and Moule (2006) suggest.

1. Identify a problem from practice and turn it into a specific question.
2. Find the best available evidence that relates to the question, usually by systematically searching the literature.
3. Appraise the evidence.
4. Identify the best evidence alongside the patient's needs and preferences.
5. Evaluate the effect of applying the evidence.

Stage 1 reflects the assessment process in nursing during which the problem to be addressed is identified and framed. Stages 2, 3 and 4 involve a conscientious and explicit planning phase during which the evidence that will underpin the plan is identified and assessed, and the patient's circumstances and preferences are accounted for. This is followed by the implementation of the plan, and the evaluation of the effectiveness of what has been done in the final stage of the nursing process and stage 5 of Hek and Moule's (2006) framework.

What is apparent from all these definitions and the application of the nursing process is that EBP is a framework for action and not academic debate and, as such, it places EBP squarely at the heart of nursing practice.

Which definition of EBP do you best identify with? Why? Do you think that this might change as you become more experienced as a nurse? Using the information presented in this section and your own experience to date, write your own definition of evidence-based practice.

As this activity is based on your own observations, there is no outline answer at the end of the chapter.

Hierarchies of evidence

This consideration of what evidence-based nursing practice is leads to an important question: if we are to evaluate the research evidence, how do we know which form of research evidence is best and consequently what we should do in practice?

Answering the question 'Which form of research evidence is best?' requires us to do two things. First, we need to understand which forms of evidence are regarded as the strongest. Second, we need to be able to evaluate individual pieces of research, identifying their strengths and weaknesses, and thereby coming to some conclusion about how good the individual piece of research is. Information on how to address this second step will be covered in more detail in Chapters 3 and 4. Here we will turn our attention to the first step.

As with the definitions of EBP there is little agreement between different professions and individual practitioners as to what constitutes good evidence. This may be surprising to the novice nurse who assumes that everyone knows what they are doing and why they are doing it. In order to understand why there are differences in opinion it is worth remembering that there are many different types of question that arise in nursing practice, and that these relate not only to the provision of specific care but also to how the care is experienced and the relationships between individuals giving and receiving care (see Chapters 3 and 4 for the types of research that are used to answer specific questions from practice). For now we should consider what is termed the hierarchy of evidence, more often presented as the hierarchy of research evidence.

Hierarchies of evidence give the practitioner and researcher alike some insight into the perceived worth of individual approaches to research. The classic hierarchy of research evidence is given in Table 1.1. It takes account only of **quantitative research** methods and does not allow for **qualitative research** methods or clinical experience or opinion.

Polit and Beck (2008, p ii) present a perhaps more useful hierarchy of evidence. This gives some weighting to evidence that takes account of qualitative research as a source of evidence as well as valuing experience and practice expertise and other evidence that is not research based (see Table 1.2). This hierarchy is more in line with the concept of evidence that is presented in this book.

Table 1.1: Example of a classic hierarchy of research evidence

	Level	Description
Strongest	1	Meta analyses and systematic reviews – reviews of multiple research reports and the statistics within them.
	2	Randomised controlled trials with definitive results – clinical trials that involve a new intervention that is assessed against another established intervention or no intervention at all and that show a definite result.
	3	Randomised controlled trials with non-definitive results – clinical trials which involve a new intervention which is assessed against another established intervention or no intervention at all which show a probable result.
	4	Prospective cohort studies/outcomes studies – long-term follow-up studies of large groups of people usually in their natural setting.
	5	Case-control studies – backward-looking studies that demonstrate associations between causes of disease and diseases or other causes and effects.
	6	Cross-sectional studies – studies undertaken in one period in time that measure potential cause and effect simultaneously.
Weakest	7	Case reports – clinical reports of individual episodes of care.

Based on the work of Petticrew and Roberts (2003).

Table 1.2: Polit and Beck's hierarchy of research evidence

	Level	Description
Strongest	1	a) Systematic review of randomised controlled trials (RCTs); b) systematic review of non-randomised trials – reviews of clinical experiments that are undertaken using: i) comparable groups; or ii) non-comparable groups.
	2	a) Single RCT; b) single non-randomised trial – i) one experimental clinical study; ii) one non-experimental clinical study.
	3	Systematic review of correlational/observational studies – reviews of studies that examine associations between causes and effects.
	4	Single correlational/observational study – one study that examines associations between causes and effects.
	5	Systematic review of descriptive/qualitative/physiologic studies – reviews of studies that only describe an event or experience or that measure individual biological variables.
	6	Single descriptive/qualitative/physiologic study – studies that only describe an event or experience or that measure individual biological variables.
Weakest	7	Opinions of authorities/expert committees – collections of the understanding and interpretations of people who are experienced in a given area.

Based on the work of Polit and Beck (2008).

| Activity 1.7 | Critical thinking |

> The NMC's generic standard for competence for Nursing practice and decision making states that: *All practice should be informed by the best available evidence and comply with local and national guidelines* (NMC, 2010, p17). Do you think that either of the hierarchies of evidence presented above enables you to do this?
>
> *There are some possible answers and thoughts at the end of the chapter.*

Hierarchies of evidence give the busy nurse some idea as to the level of trust they should place in an individual research methodology or review paper. What hierarchies don't do is answer questions about the quality of an individual piece of research (see Chapters 3 and 4) nor do they give any indication as to how to deal with an individual patient or clinical question. This is because not all research undertaken using strong research methodologies is itself good quality and because we cannot assume that the findings of a piece of research will apply to all patients who are broadly similar to those involved in the research.

In Chapter 2 issues of the identification of sources of research evidence are addressed in some detail. It is perhaps sufficient at this stage to have made the point that not all evidence is regarded as equal and that we should be aware that value judgements need to be made when thinking about the types of research evidence we choose to inform our nursing practice. We should also remember that not all evidence for nursing practice is gained from research and that there are elements of experience and reflection that also need to be accounted for, as we shall see in Chapter 5. We must also be aware that nursing is a person-centred activity and as such the application of evidence must take into account issues of policy, resources, expertise and the individual patient's situation and personal preferences.

Advancing the meaning of evidence

Typically, the greatest impacts on individual nursing practice are the clinical lessons learnt as students, and indeed, once qualified, the lessons learnt from our nursing and other professional peers. Prior to the explosion of evidence-based practice, the ward sister and the matron dictated the ways in which the nurses worked in their departments and on their wards. This 'sister knows best' working ethos still has a pervasive impact on contemporary nursing practice.

What you learn in the classroom, away from practice, often seems remote and unrelated to the realities of high turn-over, stressful nursing practice (Johnson and Ratner, 1997). Sometimes lessons learnt appear to be right in the classroom, but lose their appeal in the cold light of the practice environment. At other times it is easier to choose not to discuss or implement such lessons in order to avoid 'rocking the boat' or appearing to be a troublemaker – you might think it is perhaps best to wait until you are in charge to implement what you know to be right. The conflict between what we 'know' and what we do is a source of anxiety for many nurses and student nurses.

In part, this book lays down a challenge to all nurses, including students, to think about the ethics of what they do and how they do it. It challenges us not only to know what is right but also to practise in a way that is justifiable.

Clearly, this is a hard thing to ask of any nurse, let alone a student nurse. The question remains, however: if you would want to know the rationale for what someone is doing to you, why would you not provide a rationale for the care that you are providing to someone else?

This chapter has so far established that EBP is not an exclusively research-driven ideal but more a way of working and questioning, and drawing on sources of knowledge to continuously evolve practice. We have demonstrated that EBP is important for a number of very good reasons and we have come to some conclusions about what EBP is.

It is important at this point to say that there are a number of skills you can learn and attitudes you can adopt in order to develop EBP in your own practice. Unlike most books on evidence-based practice, this book seeks to explore and develop the skills that you need to continue to develop as a nurse who practises in an evidence-driven, patient-focused manner. In order to develop these skills you need to recognise the influences on your thinking and learning, and hence on the way in which you practise. Common influences on how you practise include: what you have been taught in your training; research you have read; experiences you have had; experience of others that you have listened to (including those of patients, nurses and other professionals); local and national policies; pressure from managers; and ethical considerations and social norms.

With all of these influences on your practice it is necessary that you learn to treat each situation as a learning experience; that is, that you are willing to learn from and apply learning to each new situation you encounter. This learning is not just about believing what you are told or what you read; it is about being critical about what you learn and experience, appraising it, considering its usefulness and seeing how it marries up with what you already know (or think you know).

One famous nursing theorist, Carper (1978), identified four ways of 'knowing' in nursing. She labelled these empirical, aesthetic, ethical and personal knowledge (an explanation of each of these is given in Table 1.3). Taken together, Carper suggests that these sources of knowledge give us the 'evidence' on which to base nursing practice.

We have established that there are a number of important influences on the way in which nursing is practised and that there are a range of forms of knowledge that might be used to inform nursing practice. What is needed now is a scheme by which we can draw all these elements together and make sense of not only sources of evidence but also influences on nursing practice.

Developing as an evidence-based nurse

Brechin (2000, p25) presents three pillars for what she calls 'critical practice', and these are presented in Table 1.4. These pillars are tools that the nurse can employ to develop an inclusive model of practice, one that recognises the need to want to do what is best for

Table 1.3: Carper's ways of 'knowing' in nursing practice

Way of knowing	Meaning
Empirical knowledge	Knowledge found in textbooks or journal papers that is derived from research and that is provable.
Aesthetic knowledge	Subjective and unique knowledge that requires interpretation, creativity, empathy, understanding and valuing. It is knowledge that feels and looks right.
Ethical knowledge	Knowledge based on systems of belief and moral codes of conduct.
Personal knowledge	Knowledge that arises out of experience as sympathy, empathy and understanding.

Based on the work of Carper (1978).

the patient while acting in a manner that respects and includes all the individuals involved, especially the patient. These pillars, or ways of working, require that even as the nurse becomes more practised and knowledgeable in what they do, they take on board and adapt this knowledge in the light of new information, evidence and individual circumstances.

Brechin's pillars tell us something about the sort of person that is needed and the attitude to care that is required of the evidence-based nurse. They support the notions that were advanced earlier in the chapter – that becoming an evidence-based nurse is about making a positive difference and that this difference has to be made in conjunction with our patients and other staff.

Barnett (2000) claims that professional life now requires more than the handling of mere complexity (i.e. managing overwhelming data and theories). It is also about handling multiple frames of reference – a condition he calls supercomplexity. Supercomplexity might arise in nursing practice when the nurse is required to pay attention not only to the realities of a patient's condition and its treatment (Carper's empirical knowledge) but also to the patient's circumstances and wishes (aesthetic knowledge), the policies and practices of the hospital, their own values and moral codes (ethical knowledge) and their own previous experiences of delivering care to someone in a similar position or with the same disease (personal knowledge).

Table 1.4: Brechin's pillars of critical practice

Pillar	What this might mean	Example
Forging relationships	Working with others.	Being open and honest in communication.
Seeking to empower others	Giving back control.	Seeking to support patient choices.
Making a difference	Improving something.	Playing a part in helping someone recover from illness.

Based on the work of Brechin (2000).

Barnett (2000) asserts that the main teaching task of a higher education institute should not just be to transmit knowledge but should be to develop in students the attributes appropriate to conditions of supercomplexity. It is the intention of this book to signpost and start to explore some of these attributes and present you, the reader, with options for self-development that will enable you to embrace a life of learning, development and evidenced care giving.

In order to achieve this state whereby one is able to function within supercomplex systems, Barnett claims that you must embrace three dimensions of being: knowledge, self-identity and action. These three elements of making sense of a complex workplace reflect quite well the central arguments of this book and this chapter – that evidence-based practice is about:

- knowledge (perhaps research based);
- working with others (especially patients) and
- the delivery of care (that is, EBP is about action and not just words).

A model of evidence-based nursing

The model of evidence-based nursing on which this book is based is one of informed nursing action delivered with an understanding and appreciation of the complexity not only of the information associated with the medical management of a patient but also of the complex nature of human interaction, beliefs and ethics. Figure 1.1 presents some of the influences on the nurse practising in an evidence-based manner. It shows some of the attributes and skills that need to be developed in order to become an evidence-based nurse and illustrates that all action has to take account of ethical and moral practice.

Figure 1.1: The influences on and dispositions of an evidence-based nurse

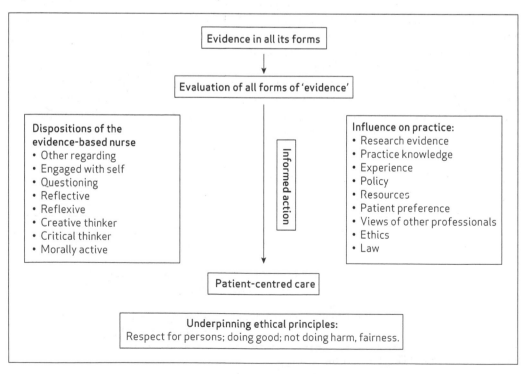

The rest of the book is given over to examining and explaining these various skills, sources and knowledge. Taken together, they form one proposal for how you might develop to become, and continue to be, an evidence-based nurse.

Activity 1.9   *Critical thinking*

Adopting the questioning approach to practice (see Figure 1.1), which embraces and juggles many seemingly competing sources of knowledge, while adopting some positive personal attributes or dispositions (characteristics) advocated in Figure 1.1, is seemingly a hard task. There appear to be a large number of things that the nurse needs to do in order to engage with this model. This is certainly true.

Now reflect on your own personal and professional behaviours and orientations to nursing practice. For example, why did you become a nurse and what was it that you thought you might achieve by taking on this role? Which of the attributes do you already possess? Which of these attributes would you like to develop? Can you see any connections between the dispositions? Are there some that you think complement each other?

There are some possible answers and thoughts at the end of the chapter.

C H A P T E R   S U M M A R Y

You may have formed the impression during your training or time on the wards that evidence-based practice was really only a term that academics used to disguise modules about research. The main message of the book is that evidence-based practice is about using various forms of information – not just research – to guide and develop practice.

In this chapter we have seen that identifying and adopting evidence for practice is a multi-stage process that requires discovering sources of potential knowledge and then asking questions about the quality of the information found.

We have identified and demonstrated that EBP is about action and not just words. It is about what we do and how we can know that what we are doing in clinical practice is the right thing to do. We have seen that evidence takes many forms and that there are a number of skills and attitudes to learning that need to be adopted by the nurse in order to support the creation and adoption of evidence-based practice.

This chapter has established that nurses need to identify high-quality sources of knowledge for practice and that they need to take account of the quality of the information that these sources present. It has shown that to be a successful evidence-based nurse, one has to engage in lifelong learning and adopt a questioning approach to one's practice. This chapter has discussed the need to involve the patient and other professionals in decision making about the patient's care and the fact that research evidence alone does not always provide sufficient grounds on which to base clinical decision making and action.

Activities: brief outline answers

Activity 1.2: Reflection (page 7)

There is a clear link between our ability as nurses to explain to our patients what we are doing and our ability to explain why. All too often nurses are involved in care but do not understand the rationale behind what they are doing. This will mean that the information passed to patients (in which I include myself and family members) is about what is going to happen and not why or how this will help. Over the last 20 or 30 years there has been a growing acceptance among nurses that this is no longer an acceptable way to practise and that as nurses we need to be able to justify what we do in practice to – and, indeed, with – our patients and clients.

Activity 1.4: Critical thinking (page 8)

The 'four principles' approach to ethics might suggest that evidence-based practice is about doing good (beneficence) by selecting the right evidence for the care of an individual and in so doing avoiding doing harm (non-maleficence) by choosing the least bad course of action. In the process of selecting a course of action with a patient – rather than for a patient – the nurse has shown respect for patient autonomy. By always supporting their patient's wishes the nurse might be said to be acting fairly and showing justice in their actions. The other school of ethical thought that might inform practice is that of consequentialism (doing things that have the best outcomes). The nurse might select a course of action with their patient that is perceived to have the highest probability of achieving the desired outcome of care.

Activity 1.5: Critical thinking (page 9)

Evidence-based practice is important for nursing for a number of very important reasons. These include:

- accountability to our professional body;
- potential for good quality outcomes of care;
- professionalism;
- governance;
- good use of resources;
- moral and ethical reasons;
- improvement of clients' lives;
- aid to planning effective interventions.

Activity 1.7: Critical thinking (page 13)

The hierarchies of evidence allow us to make judgements about the likely usefulness of competing forms of evidence in our planning and delivery of care. They suggest quite strongly that some forms of evidence are better than others at informing what we might do and how we do it. Clearly, as with all elements of evidence-based practice, the findings of research need to be interpreted alongside the patient's situation, the skills and resources available, and the patient's preference.

Activity 1.9: Critical thinking (page 17)

What appears clear from the dispositions of the evidence-based nurse is that there are a number of important links between some attributes, such as: 'other regarding' and 'morally active'; 'questioning' and 'critical thinker'; and 'engaged with self' and 'reflective'.

The development of a more structured approach to questioning, as derived from critical thinking, will also feed into the individual nurse becoming more questioning in general; while adopting a more other focused way of thinking will certainly add something to the nurse's ability to think morally and ethically.

It is probably true that you entered nursing to make a difference to the lives of patients and that you are reading this book because you think it might enhance your ability to do so. This demonstrates that you may already have attributes that include being 'other regarding', questioning and reflective. Learning to see how all of these dispositions come together to create and enhance evidence-based practice is therefore only a matter of consciously engaging with the process of consolidating, developing and exploring the links between attributes that you already have while being open to cultivating new attributes to complement them.

Knowledge review

Now that you have completed the chapter, how would you rate your knowledge of the following topics?

	Good	Adequate	Poor
1. Why EBP is important.			
2. What EBP is.			
3. The attributes and skills that an evidence-based nurse might need.			
4. How EBP contributes to patient care.			

Where you're not confident in your knowledge of a topic, what will you do next?

Further reading

Gerish, K and **Lacey, A** (eds) (2006) *The research process in nursing* (5th ed.). Oxford: Blackwell (especially Chapter 31).
This chapter examines what evidence-based practice might look like.

Gomm, R and **Davies C** (eds) (2000) *Using evidence in health and social care.* London: Sage (especially Chapters 1 and 7).
These chapters examine the different ways in which we can know things and how we can get evidence into practice.

Hek, G and **Moule, P** (2006) *Making sense of research: an introduction for health and social care practitioners* (3rd ed.). London: Sage (especially Chapters 1 and 2).
These chapters explore the role of research in EBP and also the nature of knowledge for nursing practice in its many forms.

Parahoo, K (2006) *Nursing research: principles, process and issues* (2nd ed.). London: Palgrave Macmillan (especially Chapters 1 and 2).
These chapters explore the role of research in nursing practice and the nature of knowledge for nursing practice.

Useful websites

http://clinicalevidence.bmj.com/ceweb/index.jsp This is an interesting, very clinically orientated website that examines the evidence around a variety of medical conditions and is regularly updated.

www.dh.gov.uk/en/Healthcare/Coronaryheartdisease/Nationalserviceframework/index.htm The website for the National Service Framework for Coronary Heart Disease is worth looking at to see who is involved in drawing up the framework and how it is presented as a guide to good practice in this area.

www.dh.gov.uk/en/Healthcare/Diabetes/index.htm The website for the National Service Framework for Diabetes is worth looking at to see who is involved in drawing up the framework and how it is presented as a guide to good practice in this area.

www.nice.org.uk This is the website for the National Institute for Health and Clinical Excellence where you might examine some of the criteria NICE uses in order to evaluate medications and interventions for clinical practice.

Chapter 2

Sources of knowledge for evidence-based care

Kay Hutchfield

NMC Standards for Pre-registration Nursing Education (2010)

This chapter will address the following competencies:

Domain 1: Professional values

7. All nurses must be responsible and accountable for keeping their knowledge and skills up to date through continuing professional development. They must aim to improve their performance and enhance the safety and quality of care through evaluation, supervision and appraisal.

Domain 3: Nursing practice and decision-making

1. All nurses must use up-to-date knowledge and evidence to assess, plan, deliver and evaluate care, communicate findings, influence change and promote health and best practice. They must make person-centred, evidence-based judgments and decisions, in partnership with others involved in the care process, to ensure high quality care. They must be able to recognise when the complexity of clinical decisions requires specialist knowledge and expertise, and consult or refer accordingly.

8. All nurses must provide educational support, facilitation skills and therapeutic nursing interventions to optimise health and wellbeing. They must promote self-care and management whenever possible, helping people to make choices about their healthcare needs, involving families and carers where appropriate, to maximise their ability to care for themselves.

10. All nurses must evaluate their care to improve clinical decision-making, quality and outcomes, using a range of methods, amending the plan of care, where necessary, and communicating changes to others.

Domain 4: Leadership, management and team working

2. All nurses must systematically evaluate care and ensure that they and others use the findings to help improve people's experience and care outcomes and to shape future services.

Essential Skills Clusters

This chapter will address the following ESCs:

Cluster: Care, compassion and communication

1. As partners in the care process, people can trust a newly registered graduate nurse to provide collaborative care based on the highest standards, knowledge and competence.

By entry to the register:

8. Demonstrates clinical confidence through sound knowledge, skills and understanding relevant to field.

Cluster: Organisational aspects of care

10. People can trust the newly registered graduate nurse to deliver nursing interventions and evaluate their effectiveness against the agreed assessment and care plan.

By the second progression point:

4. Actively seeks to extend knowledge and skills using a variety of methods in order to enhance care delivery.
15. People can trust the newly registered graduate nurse to safely delegate to others and to respond appropriately when a task is delegated to them.

By entry to the register:

5. Recognises and addresses deficits in knowledge and skill in self and others and takes appropriate action.

Chapter aims

After reading this chapter, you will be able to:

- identify various sources of knowledge for nursing practice;
- understand how to undertake basic online searches for literature;
- identify the level of reliability of sources of knowledge;
- demonstrate awareness of the sources policy relating to health in the UK.

Introduction

Nurses are required to provide the best quality care for people seeking help or support for their healthcare needs. To do this they are expected to be aware of current research, policies, standards, guidance and recommendations for their area of professional practice, so that the care they provide is *evidence-based*. This chapter will consider the skills needed to search for, find and evaluate the quality of the sources of evidence needed to support academic work and professional practice. It will discuss the various sources/resources that can be used to access reliable information and provide some frameworks for judging the quality of the information found.

There are many web addresses within this chapter as well as a number of searching strategies and issues identified. Rather than present activities for you to undertake, as we do in the rest of the book, you are invited to access some of the websites, search engines and other resources identified here. You might like to do a number of things along the way such as trying some searches and gathering data either on a topic of interest or for your next assignment. It might be wise to bookmark many of the sources, as you may wish to return to them in the future.

Skills needed to search for evidence

When searching online sources of evidence it is important to be organised and to plan your search for information so that you make effective use of the time you have available to you. A well-planned search is more likely to be successful in finding the information you need and will reduce the likelihood of you being sidetracked looking at information that may be only distantly connected to your topic.

All search strategies requires six elements to be successful:

1. selection of a topic;
2. identification of key words (the words that best describe the topic);
3. focusing the search;
4. extending or refining the search;
5. identification of appropriate sources;
6. keeping an accurate record of the search.

Step 1: Selection of a topic

Whatever the topic for your search you will need to have some knowledge of the subject in order to move on to Step 2. In practice, this information will be accessed through patients' notes, discussion with your mentor, patients or other healthcare colleagues. In university the module handbook, bibliography, lectures and seminars will all provide you with some key words with which to begin your search.

Step 2: Identification of key words

Key words are similar to the words you might find in the index of a book. In your nursing textbooks the authors have provided you with an index so you can easily locate the precise piece of information you need using a key word. When searching the internet the 'index' of key words will be vast. For example, entering 'communication' into the commercial search engine Google™ will result in excess of 260 million hits, which is an impossible amount of material to read though to find the specific communication information you are seeking. This illustrates the need for you to be as precise with your key words as possible when searching the web to reduce the number of 'hits' to a more manageable number.

Identifying key words may be a quick and simple task if the topic is one with which you are familiar. Taking five minutes to jot down single words associated with the topic may be all that is needed for you to produce a comprehensive list of key words. If the topic is new and unfamiliar to you, however, the task of identifying key words may be more of a challenge. In this situation you could begin by reading through course information or recommended literature in your module/programme bibliographies to help you identify key words. Alternatively, you can use a thesaurus such as the one available at www.thesaurus.com. Entering your initial key word into this online thesaurus can help to expand your list of key words and increase the chances of finding relevant material. Using some of these ideas should enable you not only to increase your list of key words but also to identify some key words that have the same or similar meanings. However, you will need to be aware that some general resources such as an online thesaurus may not always use words in the same way that they are meant in the nursing or academic sense.

At this early stage of a search other internet sources can also be useful to expand the number of key words. Wikipedia is a free online encyclopaedia that can prove a useful starting point for identifying additional key words (**http://en.wikipedia.org/wiki/Main_Page**). Returning to our example of communication, Wikipedia provides a section on communication that includes definitions and is subdivided under content headings. These headings may prove useful as an initial source of information, for refining your search of professional specific websites and databases. Wikipedia should, however, be used with caution, as it is only weakly peer reviewed – that is, the quality and correctness of the entries has not been verified by other experts in the area. For this reason, you are likely to find that your university teaching staff will not accept Wikipedia as a reference source. Use it for identifying key words and background information only.

Once you have identified a number of key words it is possible to construct a spider diagram or mind map that enables you to identify the breadth of the subject and the factors associated with it. The next stage is to create a focus for your search so that you search only for information most relevant to your needs.

Step 3: Focusing the search

If we take abuse of elderly adults as a broad topic area, you need to consider what key words from your mind map of the topic are most likely to result in the information you need, for example, if you are interested in recognising the signs of physical abuse in elderly people.

You then need to identify a list of key words that focuses your search on this area of abuse. This list might look something like this: elderly, adult, abuse, physical, signs, symptoms.

At this stage it is important to add words to your list that may have similar or the same meaning as your initial key words (synonyms), such as: aged, pensioner, vulnerable, injury. As you begin to find relevant information you will be able to expand your list of key words and became more precise.

Step 4: Extending or refining the search

Once you have produced a number of key words relevant to your search you need to consider how these might be combined to refine your search further when you are using electronic sources, e.g. commercial search engines, information gateways, library catalogues or databases. The words 'AND, OR' are the most common words used for this process. These words (AND/OR) are called Boolean operators and are named after a mathematician, George Boole.

Concept summary: Boolean operators

'AND' allows you to *limit* your search for information to two or more subjects by developing search statements. For example, if you want to do a search about the physical abuse of children, then your key words would be 'abuse', 'physical' and 'children' and combined would be 'abuse AND physical AND children'. The search results will include only results that include all three key words.

'OR' allows you to *broaden* your search for information where several different terms may be used for the same thing. For example, 'elderly OR elder OR older person OR pensioner'. By using all these terms, a wider range of material can be accessed that relates to the elderly. By inserting the word 'OR' the search will ensure the information found is about all the key words entered, but in this case not all the material found will include all the key words used.

Not all search engines have the facility to refine searches in this way and so reducing the number of hits to a manageable number may not be easy or possible. Look at the search engine help page to find hints and tips on searching in particular resources.

Concept summary continued

'NOT' is another Boolean operator that can be used to limit a search. For example, you want to find information about physical abuse but find a lot of information on neglect is included. To refine your search you could add 'NOT neglect' to exclude this term from your search.

Further information on refining your search can be found in another book in this series *Information skills for nursing students.*

Step 5: Identification of appropriate sources

This section provides a general discussion on sources, which is developed in more detail in the 'Sources of evidence' section of this chapter.

The resources available through your university or hospital library will generally be the most reliable for academic and nursing practice purposes and will have been recommended by academic staff as appropriate for your programme. Making decisions about the reliability of other sources you regularly access is an important skill to develop.

You will be familiar with finding out information from a range of sources such as newspapers, radio, television news and documentaries or by searching the web using commercial search engines such as Google. However, you will need to learn about new resources when you join a nursing programme. Learning how to use them will take time and effort, but will benefit you by enabling you to access sources of information that you will use throughout your university studies and professional career and will save you time in the long term.

This does not mean that you cannot use commercial search engines, blogs or Wikipedia to support your studies, but they do need to be used with caution. This is because anyone can publish on the 'world wide web', so it is possible that some material may be inaccurate, out of date or even deliberately misleading. If using these sources, care must be taken to consider issues of quality.

Theory

There are a number of questions that you can ask about the quality of various sources of information even before you read what they contain. While this is not an exhaustive list, some of the key questions include the following.

- Can you identify the author of the information?
- What qualifications do they have and can you find any other information about them on the internet that would confirm they are an expert in the field they are writing about?
- When was the material written? This is often difficult to establish on many websites.
- What evidence do they provide to support any statements or claims?
- What type of website is the information on? Is it a commercial site that is trying to encourage you to spend money on their products or is it a non-profit making organisation such as a charity?
- Is it an academic website produced by a university or other academic institution?

Table 2.1: Understanding URLs

Elements of URL for Google, **www.google.co.uk**	**www.google.co.uk** is the domain name and has several elements.
www.	www. stands for **w**orld **w**ide **w**eb (not all sites have this).
google.	Google is the name of the organisation that has exclusive rights to use that domain name.
co.	This part of the domain tells you what type of organisation is publishing the website. In this case .co or .com tells you that Google is a commercial organisation. Sites such as this one make a profit through selling products and services and/or through advertising.
.uk	This element tells you it is a UK-based website.

In order to establish the type of website you are accessing you need to be familiar with the information available from the URL (Uniform Resource Locator) or web address. Google is an example of a website you are likely to be familiar with. The URL for Google is **www.google.co.uk**. Table 2.1 provides information about each element of the URL that will tell you what sort of website you have accessed.

When accessing any website, the type of organisation publishing the site is particularly important to note. UK schools, colleges and universities will have ac.uk at the end of the URL; government organisations will have .gov.uk and the NHS will have nhs.uk. You should also be aware that some websites that carry the .uk suffix may not be based in the UK and you will need to exercise judgement about how much faith you can place in their contents.

Step 6: Keeping an accurate record of your search

Before you begin your search there is one more task to consider, and that is keeping a record of your search. Keeping a record of *what* key words you used, *when and where* you have used them and *what* information you found is an essential part of any search strategy. Keeping accurate records of your search will save you a great deal of time and avoid the frustration of losing track of the sources of useful information. Sometimes you may be able to keep a record by printing out or saving an electronic search record.

Sources of evidence

Table 2.2 contains some examples of the type of sources you will be expected to use to support your assignments and your professional practice. Intute is accessible at **www.intute.ac.uk** and offers an outline of the type of professional resources that have been summarised in the table.

It is *essential* you begin to learn to use some bibliographic databases, electronic journals and information gateways to ensure you can access material of good quality from a range of sources that will enable you to keep up to date with current practice. University libraries will normally offer workshops and online tutorials on how to use these professional sources of information. Make good use of these resources so you continue to develop your searching skills over the course of your programme.

Table 2.2: Sources of information to support professional practice

Publications from key organisations	For example, Department of Health, World Health Organization, National Patient Safety Agency.
Electronic journals	These are becoming increasingly available; however, many require subscription. Remember to find out what e-journals your university subscribes to in your subject area.
Bibliographic databases	The Cochrane Library and Pubmed offer free access to a range of evidence-based information.
	Other bibliographic databases such as CINAHL (Cumulative Index of Nursing and Allied Health Literature) and ASSIA (Applied Social Sciences Index and Abstracts) require a subscription and may be available through your university library.
Information gateways	These specialist websites are often organised under subject headings to provide access to specific web-based information. Intute is one example.
Library catalogues	These catalogues list all the print items owned by the library.
Professional organisations	For example, the Nursing and Midwifery Council and the Royal College of Nursing are two key nursing organisations that provide information to guide and direct nursing practice.
News and media	BBC news:health and Guardian.co.uk:health (**www.bbc.co.uk/health**) are two examples of sources of media-generated health information.
Web 2 technology	Blogs, wikis, podcasts and video sharing are becoming increasingly popular mechanisms for sharing information. However, these sites must be used with caution as the reliability of the information cannot always be established.

Source: adapted from material available on Intute, 2010.

The next sections review sources that are relevant to nursing. The review will begin with some sources that may already be familiar to you but have to be used with caution as the evidence they provide cannot always be authenticated.

Wikipedia

Wikipedia is a very convenient source of initial information and may be one with which you are already familiar.

> *Wikipedia is a . . . web-based, free-content encyclopedia project based . . . Wikipedia is written collaboratively by largely anonymous internet users who write without pay. Anyone with internet access can write and make changes to Wikipedia articles.*
>
> Wikipedia, 2010

Wikipedia is quick and easy to use, and as a first source of information it can be a useful introduction to a new topic. However, it is often difficult to identify the author/co-authors of material on this site and therefore raises questions regarding reliability. Anyone can publish anonymously on this site, and as it is only weakly peer-reviewed, errors or malicious entries may remain accessible before they are corrected or removed. Therefore, when using Wikipedia as a source as evidence it is essential that you use additional, more reliable sources of evidence to confirm the reliability of the information you have found.

It is important to note that the need to be cautious about the sources of information you use to generate evidence for your nursing practice is as strong as the need to learn the skills of critical appraisal and research critiquing, which are discussed in other chapters in this book.

Google Scholar

If you are familiar with using Google to find information, you may initially feel more comfortable beginning with this source. Like the generic Google search engine, Google Scholar™ is a free online search tool that provides a search of scholarly literature from a range of sources such as theses, books and articles.

Unlike Google, Google Scholar allows you to undertake a more precise search. Select 'Advanced Scholar Search', as this not only allows you to be specific about the key words you use but also allows you to search for specific authors or to limit your search by year of publication. Google Scholar also offers advanced scholar search tips that help you make the most of this resource.

The disadvantage of using Google Scholar is that it will often only provide you with an abstract of the journal articles you find, and there is often a cost to access the full text. However, you may be able to access the full text article through your university library if your university subscribes to the journal in which the article is published (this may include online access using your university library account). If this is not the case, your library may offer an interlibrary loan system for a limited number of requests and so you may still be able to access the full text through this process.

Key organisations

Key organisations such as the Department of Health (DH) can be accessed through a generic search engine such as Google. Once on the DH site it is reasonable to assume that the information it contains is reliable and based on credible evidence.

Department of Health (www.dh.gov.uk)

The Department of Health publishes many documents that provide policy, standards, recommendations and guidance that are relevant to nursing and healthcare in the UK in general. The 'Health care' page provides links to all healthcare publications and to the National Service Frameworks (NSFs) that provide standards for care in a range of areas, including children and maternity care, coronary heart disease, mental health and diabetes. Understanding the policy context of care is an important element of the evidence-based nursing process, and in the UK the DH website is the most important source for these.

The DH website also provides links to current news and updates and access to the NHS Evidence search portal that *provides rapid access to information for everyone working in health and social care* (NHS Evidence in Health and Social Care, 2009).

National Institute for Health and Clinical Excellence (NICE) (www.nice.org.uk)

NICE is an independent organisation responsible for providing national guidance on promoting good health and preventing ill health. It provides details of the latest evidence-based guidelines, guidance and implementation and quality initiatives. It is a valuable source of clinical guidelines for nurses and other health professionals on a wide range of health topics. The processes that it uses to generate the guidelines and guidance is worth looking at as it represents what is considered by many to be good practice in evidence-based healthcare.

NHS Institute for Innovation and Improvement (www.institute.nhs.uk)

The NHS Institute for Innovation and Improvement is part of the Department of Health and is specifically focused on developing and disseminating new ways of working, new technology as well as developing leadership in healthcare. It provides practical frameworks for the improvement of the quality of care.

NHS National Patient Safety Agency (www.npsa.nhs.uk)

This agency has three distinct sections with the National Reporting and Learning Service section providing information that can improve patient care and safety. The site has a range of resources, including teaching resources designed to improve risk management in practice.

Information gateways

Intute (www.intute.ac.uk)

At the time of writing Intute is being updated regularly, but from July 2011 it may just be maintained and not necessarily added to. Intute is a web-based resource that is organised by university subject specialists into subject headings. Each subject heading provides a brief description of each of the websites included. This site is an information gateway that includes only the sites most relevant to the subject headings, and is designed to make it easier to find subject-specific information. It is not a source of academic papers or journal articles.

Intute identifies government-based sites such as the Department of Health, but it also identifies websites that are service-user focused and provides information for patients and carers. These are often useful sites for novice nurses to gain an insight into the way in which illness and disease impact on patients' lives, before progressing on to more academic sources of information. As discussed elsewhere in the book, understanding the patient experience of care is an important aspect of becoming an evidence-based nurse.

NHS libraries

NHS Evidence: Health Information Resources

As a nurse on a university programme you can gain free access to the NHS Evidence: Health Information Resources (formerly known as the National Library for Health).

NHS Evidence incorporates some of the key components from the National Library for Health, enhancing and providing the latest functionality. In addition

NHS Evidence is developing an accreditation process for sources of information
to provide confidence for users of health and social care information.
NHS Evidence: Health Information Resources website
(see 'Useful websites' section for address)

This excellent online resource is user friendly and specifically designed to provide access to evidence-based reviews, the National Library of Guidelines, NICE guidelines, books, journals, healthcare databases and much more. You will need to register for an account to access some of these resources.

NHS trust libraries

When you are on placements you have the opportunity to access your trust's NHS library. The trust librarians can direct you to the free resources available to you as a nursing student and any borrowing rights you may have. NHS and university librarians have a great deal of knowledge about the resources that are available to help inform both your academic and clinical work. As well as understanding what resources are available, these librarians also have in-depth knowledge of how bibliographic databases work and the commonly used key words in certain topic areas.

University libraries

Unlike public libraries, your university will have its own library website that will contain free resources purchased specifically for your programme. University websites provide you with access to information from academic sources that cannot be accessed through your public library, Google or Google Scholar. It is important to take advantage of any library workshops relating to the use of the resources that are relevant to your nursing programme.

Your university library will contain a range of books and journals on the shelves, but this is only a small proportion of the information held. However, before embarking on a discussion of the electronic sources of information available to students, it is important to remember that your programme/module tutor will provide you with a bibliography listing the core and recommended texts that they will expect you to read as part of the programme or module. You should use the reference information in the bibliographies as the first stage in your search information of the library catalogue.

Library catalogues

The library catalogue provides access to a complete listing of the books, DVDs and printed journals held by your university library. University libraries aim to provide a number of copies of all the recommended books for your module or programme, but there will be a limited number, so you may want to consider buying some key textbooks. Ask your personal tutor, module leader or programme director for guidance on which books they recommend you purchase.

When searching the library catalogue it is easy to find what you want if you know the title or author of the book. However, if you do not have this information, you need to remember that books contain a much wider range of information on a topic than a journal article and so the book title is likely to be broad rather than specific. For example, searching for 'pressure sores OR decubitus ulcers' may be too precise for the library catalogue. Searching for nursing care or tissue viability is more likely to provide an appropriate introduction to the topic within one of a textbook's chapters. You can also search the library catalogue by subject area, such as 'nursing care'.

When searching the library catalogue it is important to make a note of the classmark of the book. The classmark is a series of numbers and/or letters that enables you to locate a book on the library shelves. If the book you want is already on loan, you may find an alternative suitable book on the shelves by looking at books with a similar classmark.

Libraries also contain records of all the journals or periodicals the library subscribes to, and where they are located in the library. It is not advisable to search journals or periodicals by hand as an electronic search is a far more efficient use of time. However, if you have found a useful reference during a search on Google Scholar, you can use the library catalogue to search the list of journals held by the university to see if you can access a full-text hard copy for free. You can also search for journals by subject through the library catalogue. The library catalogue usually also holds details of video recordings, newspapers and large print books.

E-books

The ability to access electronic books or online versions of printed books is an expanding area and is likely to increase dramatically over the coming years. Searching Google Books is a simple way to see if you can view a book or chapter online for free. Many universities also have access to e-books.

Bibliographic databases

Your university has to pay for access to bibliographic databases and you will be given a user name and password that will enable you to access this resource. This may be referred to as your library account (previously known as ATHENS account).

A bibliographic database contains references to a vast range of published literature contained in journal articles, conference proceedings, reports, government publications and newspaper articles. Information is usually presented in the form of a reference and an abstract (or summary of the literature). Not all bibliographic databases provide access to the full text of all the information that is indexed. In these cases it may be necessary to record the reference and seek a full-text copy via your library's print or electronic holdings or through their interlibrary loan system.

If you have the name of a particular journal or subject area, you can search for it through your university library database to see if the full text is available. Knowing the volume and issue number of the article you wish to find will greatly increase the likelihood of finding the article you need through e-journal searching.

When using bibliographic databases it is important to use those that are the most relevant to your subject area. For nursing students CINAHL (Cumulative Index of Nursing and Allied Health Literature) and the British Nursing Index may the most useful, along with PsycINFO, which covers all aspects of psychology.

EBSCO*host* Electronic Journals Service (EJS) is one gateway to thousands of e-journals containing millions of articles from hundreds of different publishers, all on one website. This may be available to you via your university library website.

Medline includes literature relating to medicine but also includes nursing and allied health literature. ASSIA is the Applied Social Science Index and Abstracts. This database contains over 255,000 records dating back to 1987 and may be a useful source of information on a topic that has a social as well as a medical/nursing focus, for example domestic violence.

Choosing which source to search will be dependent on the topic. Use your university librarian to help you identify which sources are the most likely to contain the information you seek.

The Cochrane Centre

The UK Cochrane Centre is one of twelve centres worldwide that facilitate and co-ordinate the publication of systematic reviews of randomised controlled trials. It also provides training for contributors. To search this site, enter via the Cochrane Library webpage **www.thecochranelibrary.com/view/o/index.html**.

Systematic reviews are regarded by many as the most reliable source of evidence for practice; however, such reviews will not exist for all areas where evidence is required.

Demographic information

The Office of National Statistics is a source of demographic information related to England, Wales, Scotland and Northern Ireland.

> *[It] covers population and demographic information. It contains commentary on the latest findings, topical articles on relevant subjects such as one parent families, cohabitation, fertility differences, international demography, population estimates and projections for different groups. Illustrated with colour charts and diagrams, regularly updated statistical tables and graphs, showing trends and the latest quarterly information on: conceptions, births, marriages, divorces, internal and international migration, population estimates and projections, etc.*
>
> Home page of Office of National Statistics website
> (see 'Useful websites' section for address)

Professional bodies/organisations

Nursing and Midwifery Council

The Nursing and Midwifery Council (NMC) is the statutory body set up to regulate the nursing and midwifery profession in the UK. The NMC website (**www.nmc-uk.org**) provides access to all their standards, publications and consultations that nurses and midwives have to comply with.

The site also enables employers to check the registration status of their employees and to access information on current Fitness to Practise (FtP) hearings. The records of these hearings provide insight into the reasons why nurses may be removed from the nursing register and can make interesting reading.

The NMC website and the information it contains can be a useful source for identifying the context of care. Understanding the context of care is helpful in establishing the credibility and usefulness of evidence for practice.

Royal College of Nursing

The Royal College of Nursing (RCN) was founded in 1916. It is a membership organisation made up mainly of registered nurses, but it also includes student nurses and healthcare assistants. Its aims are to *represent nurses and nursing, promote excellence* in practice and influence healthcare policy. Services include free access to the extensive RCN library. Membership of this organisation also allows you access to their numerous publications and research. The RCN website offers guidance on professional development that includes guides to using their library services.

News and media

Newspapers and television often contain health information. These sources need to be viewed with caution as they do not always present a complete or unbiased view of health topics; however, they do provide a source of information for the general public, so keeping up to date with the content of the health pages of newspapers, news programmes and documentaries can provide an insight into the patients' perspective and expectations of healthcare provision. As discussed throughout this book, the patient view of care forms part of the evidence base of nursing care.

These sources may provide a focus for exploring a topic but should not be used as the sole source of evidence to support or change practice. Rather, they should be viewed as a motivation for a more comprehensive and academic investigation.

Blogs

The personal knowledge and experiences of patients, clients and carers have been recognised by some as a valid source of information to inform clinical practice (Rycroft-Malone et al., 2004). Such information may be gathered in a variety of ways. Patient satisfaction surveys or audits of the patient experience provide quantitative data that can be utilised to improve the quality of service provision. Other sources of information may be much more difficult to utilise.

Blogs can provide a personal commentary on a particular topic such as politics or news, or be a form of personal online diary or journal. A blog is an individual record of an experience and provides a personal, subjective perspective on a topic. This must be remembered if you use the content of a blog as evidence to support your studies. For instance, you may come across the blog of a woman who has experienced breast cancer in which she suggests that practice could be improved for such patients. In this situation it is important to remember that this 'evidence' relates to the experience of one person and so cannot be **generalised** to the experience of all patients with breast cancer. However, knowledge of a range of different patient experiences may enable you to be more sensitive to the individual responses and needs of patients with specific conditions, rather than adopting a 'one size fits all' approach, and as such will form part of your personal evidence base.

Experts

The *Oxford Concise English Dictionary* (Oxford English Dictionaries, 1996) describes an expert as 'having special skill at a task or knowledge in a subject'. It is often a combination of knowledge, experience and skill that makes us regard others as expert in nursing, and during your time as a nursing student you will meet many different experts, including expert patients and expert carers. These experts will provide some of the evidence you will use to support your practice.

When you first begin your nursing career it may seem that everyone but you is an expert. In your placement your mentor will be the expert in nursing who will guide, supervise and assess your practice. Initially, it is likely that you will take such direction with little questioning, but as you progress you will need to become less dependent on direction from others and more reliant on your own developing knowledge and expertise.

Your knowledge of theoretical perspectives will increase as the programme progresses and it will become less acceptable to just ask your mentor for information. You will be increasingly expected to have investigated topics yourself and be able to offer an evidence-based rationale for the care you deliver or to challenge the practice of others. This does not mean you should not seek expert advice, but rather you should actively seek to increase your own independent learning so that you can actively engage in professional debate and make a positive contribution to enhancing patient care.

Professional colleagues can be an invaluable source of knowledge and information (as explored in Chapter 6), but their views must not be accepted without criticism, as knowledge in healthcare is continuously developing. It is everyone's professional responsibility to keep up to date with changes so that when you become a registered nurse you have a knowledge base sufficient to support your practice.

Anecdotal evidence

Words associated with the word 'anecdotal' include 'subjective', 'untrustworthy' and 'undependable'. This would suggest that anecdotal evidence is not robust and perhaps more based on hearsay, myths and rituals than hard evidence.

The contents of a blog could be called anecdotal, and yet the subjective account of a person's experience of an illness may provide a powerful insight into the lived experiences of patients that nurses could use to enhance care. Narrative (storytelling) is increasingly being used as a means of exploring and identifying evidence (see Chapter 5), and so it would seem that in the future there needs to be further clarification of the term 'anecdotal' to ensure that useful evidence is not lost while myth and ritual are eliminated.

C H A P T E R   S U M M A R Y

This chapter has outlined how to develop a simple plan for finding information to inform your studies and your practice. It has identified and discussed some of the sources from which knowledge that may be used to form evidence for practice may be drawn.

Identifying sources of knowledge is clearly only the first step along the road to the generation of evidence for practice, but the same issues of being critical and thoughtful about the quality and nature of the sources that you use to inform your thinking will apply to all the stages of the evidence-based practice process.

Knowledge review

Now that you have completed the chapter, how would you rate your knowledge of the following topics?

	Good	Adequate	Poor
1. Identifying sources of knowledge for nursing.			
2. How to undertake basic online searches.			
3. Assessing the reliability of sources of knowledge.			
4. Identifying sources policy relating to health in the UK.			

Where you're not confident in your knowledge of a topic, what will you do next?

Further reading

Hutchfield, K (2010) *Information skills for nursing students*. Exeter: Learning Matters.
A comprehensive guide to identifying information for nursing students.

Rycroft-Malone, J (2008) Evidence-informed practice: from individual to context. *Journal of Nursing Management*, Special Issue, 16 (4): 404–8.
An interesting look at what evidence-based nursing might look like.

Useful websites

http://scholar.google.co.uk A Google website that specialises in scholarly articles, publications and academic theses from all subject areas.

www.institute.nhs.uk Website of the NHS Institute for Innovation and Improvement which seeks to support the NHS in transforming healthcare by the rapid development and dissemination of new ways of working.

www.intute.ac.uk A free online service that helps you to find the best online resources (reviewed by subject specialists) for your studies and research.

www.library.nhs.uk NHS Evidence, Health Information Resources website. Provides access to a wide range of resources and materials about health and social care.

www.nmc-uk.org Nursing and Midwifery Council (NMC) website. This is nursing and midwifery's regulatory body and the website contains policy documents and guidelines related to nursing and midwifery practice.

www.npsa.nhs.uk NHS National Patient Safety Agency website, which aims to improve safe patient care by informing, supporting and influencing the health sector.

www.statistics.gov.uk Office of National Statistics website. Provides useful population data pertaining to diseases and treatments that is of interest when describing the background to a health topic of interest.

Chapter 3

Critiquing research: the generic elements

Peter Ellis

Chapter aims

After reading this chapter, you will be able to:

*   describe the need for critical reviewing of research in health and social care;
*   describe the type of questions that can be applied to all research papers during the critiquing process;

Chapter aims continued

- demonstrate awareness of the systematic nature of the process of research critiquing;
- understand the ethical considerations that need to be taken into account when evaluating health and social care research.

Introduction

In this book we have established that it is important for nurses who wish to be truly evidence-based to be critical and analytical in their approach to the identification, reading and potential adoption into their practice of various sources of evidence. We have already indicated that an understanding of research **methodologies**, **methods** and analysis is useful in establishing the worth of **empirical** literature to inform evidence-based nursing practice.

The opportunities for every nurse to engage in clinical research are limited, and there are good reasons why this should be the case. One of these is the potential for over-whelming both practice and patients with requests to participate in research, thereby detracting from the delivery of good quality clinical care. Rather, the challenge is for nurses to engage with research as an important source of evidence to guide and inform practice. One practical mechanism for doing this is via a work-based or university journal club that might meet to identify, critique and discuss the adoption of new research findings.

Activity 3.1	Research and finding out

Get together with some of your fellow students and set up a journal club. Use this journal club to identify and share with each other your thoughts about articles that you have found that are relevant to the module that you are studying. You could even take this one step further and use an internet social networking site to discuss the articles or books you have found and what you think about them. You may be able to set up a wiki or a discussion board to which you are all able to contribute.

As this is based on your own interaction, there is no specimen answer at the end of the chapter.

Regardless of whether all nurses are able to undertake research, they should have at least a basic understanding of how research is undertaken, and what constitutes good-quality research fit to inform their practice. Being able to judge the quality of a piece of research and its applicability to our individual clinical settings and client groups is essential if we are to use it to inform what we do in a meaningful way. So as well as being able to critique research, nurses need to understand whether the research might be useful in informing practice where they work.

It is beyond the scope of this book to look in detail at the design and execution of the various forms of research used to inform nursing practice. For a detailed look at the design and undertaking of research studies in nursing practice, or to help you with a critique of a piece of research see *Understanding research for nursing students* (also in this series – other sources you may wish to use are identified at the end of this chapter).

Because there is a need to understand some general areas for critique as well as how to critique the specifics of the two main approaches to research, qualitative and quantitative methodologies, this part of the book is split into two chapters. The first chapter, the generic section, deals with critiquing elements of published research that apply to all research papers of whatever methodology. This includes the titles, authors, choice of research paradigm and the discussion and conclusions sections of the paper as well as some consideration of the ethical questions that might be asked of a published study. The next chapter will focus on specific questions to be asked of qualitative and quantitative research. Areas for critique within the next chapter include methodological choice (design), sampling, data-collection methods and analysis of the data.

Within both chapters there are some brief descriptions and critiques of elements of various research papers. Most of these papers are readily available via university or hospital-based journal subscriptions both online and on paper. Where possible, it would help your understanding of the process of research critiquing to read some of these papers in full, although this is not absolutely necessary. Chapter 2 will help you to work out how to access these papers using electronic database searches – the details of which are explored in the book *Information skills for nursing students*, also in this series.

As well as the guidance contained within these chapters there is a comprehensive critiquing framework in the appendix to Chapter 4 that can be applied to most research. This framework is in three sections: the first applies to all research, as does this chapter; the second has additional questions that apply to qualitative research (see Chapter 4); and the third has additional questions that relate to quantitative research (also in Chapter 4). You might find it useful to read both chapters while simultaneously referring to the questions contained in this framework. Because the critiquing of research is a dynamic process where a number of judgement calls need to be made, the contents of the chapters and the questions within the framework do not exactly mirror each other.

It is important to establish right from the start that critiquing in this sense is seen not merely as an activity that is used to identify weaknesses within a study but also as an activity that seeks to establish a study's strengths and therefore the degree of faith that can be placed in its findings. So, as in the rest of the book, the critical activities are seen not merely as a means to establish weakness but also as a means of identifying good-quality evidence that may subsequently be useful in the advancement of practice. Clearly, this cannot be achieved if the sole intention of the activity is to identify and discard weak research.

The format of the presentation of this and the following chapter is intended not only to help you ask the right question of the different areas of the research papers you read but also to provide you with what you might be looking for in the way of a positive answer to the question posed. The questions and guidance in these two chapters, along with the framework in the appendix to Chapter 4, can be used to provide a map for undertaking a critique of a research paper in a meaningful and straightforward manner.

While much of what you will need to ask and the sort of answers that you will be looking for is contained within these chapters and the appendix, this does not negate the need for some further reading around the methodologies and methods of the papers you may be using these chapters to help critically analyse.

If you are undertaking a critique as part of some course work, you should also refer to the assignment guidelines and ensure that you only appraise the elements of the research you are asked to critique.

Undertaking the critique

There is no single right way to approach undertaking a critique of a piece of research. There are, however, some strategies that will make the process easier for the novice to undertake and that can provide structure to the process.

Lobiondo-Wood and Haber (1998) suggest the following strategy.

- Skim read the paper to get a feel for the overall approach of the research.
- Read the paper in depth, making sure you understand each element.
- Break the study down into its component parts.
- Think about the study as a whole and consider its message.

Certainly, these are useful strategies. Highlighting important areas of the text is also useful as is drawing a simple flow diagram of the research, including the question, methodology, sample, methods, analysis, results and key discussion points, which makes referring back to the paper much easier to do and aids in the critiquing process (see Figure 3.1). A short overview of each piece of research is very helpful where you are considering critiquing a number of research papers, as you might in a review, for example.

Figure 3.1: Example overview of a randomised controlled trial

Robson, V, Dodd, S and Thomas, S (2009) Standardized antibacterial honey (MedihoneyTM) with standard therapy in wound care: randomized clinical trial. *Journal of Advanced Nursing*, 65 (3): 565–75.

↓

Aims: to compare a medical grade honey with conventional treatments on the healing rates of wounds healing by secondary intention (without surgical intervention)

↓

Methodology: Randomised controlled trial.

↓

Sample: One hospital in UK. Outpatient or inpatient. Exclude: diabetes, psychiatric illness, allergy to bees/honey, venous ulcers of less than 12 weeks, grade 1 or 4 pressure ulcers, exposed bone, tendon, muscle, malignancy in the wound, need for antibiotics for the wound in past two weeks. 105 people recruited (power calculation for 200).

↓

Methods: Baseline data collected prior to randomisation including photographs of wound and classification of wound type. Randomisation in blocks stratified (layered) by over and under forty, and wound size (greater or less than 10cm²). Full assessment of wound every two weeks until 12 weeks and then four weekly up to 24 weeks. Dressing by ward or community staff according to provided protocol – 53 conventional dressing and 52 honey.

↓

Analysis: Intention to treat (all included, even withdrawals, to reflect real life scenario). Final analysis was stratified by potential confounding factors (things that may affect result): gender and wound type. Days from randomisation to healing recorded. Days from randomisation to 50% reduction in wound size.

↓

Results: Median time to healing: 100 days (honey), 140 days (conventional) – not statistically significant (ns). Healing rate at 12 weeks: 46.2% v 34% (ns). At 24 weeks: 72.7% v 63.3% (ns). Adjusted results for age, gender, wound type and wound area (ns).

↓

Discussion: During the life of the study honey became available for wounds on prescription and was widely publicised. The study was therefore stopped prematurely as some patients and nurses wanted the honey treatment without risking being randomised to the control group. Limited amounts of other useful studies in this area to support a change in practice.

A much briefer flow diagram of such research can prove useful for gaining an overview of a single piece of research and for comparing the processes with a number of different research studies. In fact, the Consolidated Standards of Reporting Trials (CONSORT) group, who are concerned with improving the reporting of clinical trials, have created a flow diagram for this very purpose, which demonstrates how data can be downsized into manageable chunks for the purposes of review. Clearly, this template applies only to clinical trials and shows participant movement through a trial, but the idea can be adapted to suit all research methodologies and further notes can be added as required.

Activity 3.2   *Research and finding out*

Visit the CONSORT website at **www.consort-statement.org/consort-statement/ flow-diagramo/** and download a copy of the flow diagram. Take some time to look over the way in which it is present and consider how you might use and adapt it for yourself.

As this activity is based on your own considerations, there is no outline answer at the end of the chapter.

A further useful (and often overlooked) part of the process of an academic critique is the use of research resources to inform the process. This involves using books about research to highlight the processes that a research study might undertake in the ideal world. What actually happened in the study you are reviewing is then compared to these processes as part of your critique.

Of course, it is often the case that you will understand different sections in certain books better than in others, so use more than one textbook against which to compare the research that you are reading.

Theory

When undertaking an assignment as part of a course or module of study, it is usual to follow certain academic conventions. The need to follow these conventions is no different when undertaking a critique. The usual strategy when approaching this sort of work is to: define your terms (explain what a technical word means); reference the definition (to an academic text such as a research textbook); and apply the definition to the critique you are undertaking. There is then a higher probability that you understand the new terminology and that the marker understands what it is you are trying to say and is sure that you understand what it is you are saying.

Many textbooks and websites about research and evidence-based practice contain frameworks that can be used to guide the process of critiquing a research paper (see the Further reading and Useful websites sections at the end of the chapter). They point the reader in the direction of the correct questions to ask at the different stages of the review; in general, they are best used in conjunction with at least one research textbook. It is important to ascertain what types of research the frameworks are written in relation to, as some are generic (that is, they apply to all methodologies) while others are specific to either the **qualitative** or **quantitative paradigms**, and yet others relate only to individual specific methodologies. The critiquing framework presented in the appendix to Chapter 4 is both generic – it can be used to ask questions of all research methodologies – and specific – it contains paradigm-specific elements.

Generic questions

There are some questions that apply to all the research papers that you might read. These generic questions relate to some of the core decisions about the general approach to the research being undertaken, how ethically the research has been undertaken and, to a lesser extent, the title of the paper and the credentials of the authors. There are some common pitfalls and assumptions that students make when critiquing research that will be identified below, and some ideas about how to overcome these and establish the quality of the critique being undertaken.

This notion of the quality of the critique is in many respects as important as the notion of the quality of the research paper. If the idea of learning to prepare, and indeed undertaking, a research critique is to provide evidence to inform clinical practice, then the process by which this is achieved must also be robust. Clearly, this is also important for the student who is seeking to gain a good mark for a piece of course work as well!

Title

Many critiquing frameworks require the user to make decisions about the quality of some issues relating to the title of the paper being critiqued. Certainly, it is very frustrating to find that the content of a paper bears no resemblance to what appears in the title. There can also be an issue with being able to identify from a paper's title that it is a research paper rather than a review or an opinion piece.

The truth of the matter is that more often than not the authors of journal papers have limited input into the title their paper is given. The journal staff sometimes choose the title of the paper as a means of attracting potential readers to both the individual article and the journal.

Activity 3.3   *Reflection*

What strategies might you use when reading a journal paper to identify rapidly whether you are reading original research or some other type of publication such as a review or opinion paper?

There are some possible answers at the end of the chapter.

Clearly, if you are required to critique elements of a research paper such as the title as part of some coursework, then you must; ordinarily, however, it is not considered an important element of the critiquing process. As a general rule, a good title will identify the characteristics of the participants (e.g. people with diabetes), the nature of the research questions (e.g. quality of life) and the methodological approach used (e.g. phenomenology). Some titles may also include some message about the key findings of the research, although this is not always possible.

Author credentials

In essence, the author credentials are not as important as the quality of the research itself as all researchers have to start with a first paper and therefore limited publishing credentials (Coughlan et al., 2007). Checking the authors' credentials requires understanding of at least one of three main areas: their qualifications, their current work role and their previous publications.

It may be preferable for someone undertaking nursing research to have a nursing background and this may be established within the paper. Many journals do not publish authors' qualifications, however, so this is not always easily ascertained. It would therefore not be possible to critique credibility from this angle.

The author's role(s) can give a reasonable insight into what experience they have of the topic in hand – many journals publish this. Although we said that it may be preferable for nursing research to be undertaken by nurses, this certainly does not exclude research undertaken by people with other professional or academic backgrounds. Much of the knowledge base for nursing has been gained from other professional and academic disciplines, so it is common for individuals other than nurses to contribute to or undertake research that is applicable to nursing.

The third strategy that can be applied to establishing the author's credentials is to look at their publication history. This can often be achieved by finding their profile(s) (where these exist) – for example, on a university website – and where these are not available, by doing an author search on a bibliographic database to identify papers they have published on the topic of interest. A note of caution: sometimes the author with the research expertise is not the first author; for example, when a lecturer publishes work together with a research student, it may be necessary to search for more than just the first author.

The choice of research paradigm

The choice of research paradigm will depend on the type of question – or questions – that a piece of research is setting out to answer (Polit and Beck, 2006). Essentially, in health and social care (including nursing) research there are two distinct research paradigms. These paradigms represent two distinct, but not entirely separate, philosophical ways of viewing the world and asking questions. You may be familiar with the terms for these philosophical approaches: the qualitative paradigm and the quantitative paradigm.

Activity 3.4   *Reflection*

What do the words 'qualitative' and 'quantitative' mean to you? Can you identify the philosophical underpinnings of the two approaches from their names?

There are some possible answers at the end of the chapter.

Given the answers to Activity 3.4, it is apparent that the approach to answering a question arising from nursing practice will depend on the nature of the question. Questions that focus on how people experience their world, what their attitudes are and how they perceive things will sit within the qualitative paradigm and will require that qualitative methodologies and methods are used to investigate them, while questions about cause and effect and things that can be enumerated will require a quantitative research approach.

Concept summary: triangulation

Given the differences in approach to asking and answering questions, it would seem logical to expect to see research using either a qualitative or a quantitative approach to answering questions. While this is often the case, some research employs mixed methodologies and methods in order to look at a research question from more than one angle – this is called **triangulation**.

This triangulation of methodologies and methods allows the researchers not only to ask questions about *what* happens under which circumstances and *how* it happens (as in quantitative research) but also to explore *why* people behave as they do or have the beliefs and opinions that they express (as in qualitative research). For example, *quantitatively* it can be demonstrated that a diet that is high in saturated fats is bad for health. In order to address individuals' eating behaviours, however, it is first necessary to understand, using *qualitative* methods, why people make the lifestyle choices they do.

The background/introduction/literature review, which is at the start of all good research papers, will help establish the credentials of the study as a qualitative or quantitative study (Hek and Moule, 2006). A good introduction will explore the state of the literature about the topic of interest and will establish what important older (but recent) research has shown about it. Essentially, it is usual for the argument put forward in the introduction to the paper to lead the reader to the point where they can appreciate the sorts of questions that need answering about the topic of the research.

It is these questions posed in the introduction that will frame the research as either quantitative or qualitative.

Example critique: choice of paradigm

In Jones's (2003) study, which set out to *explore the perceptions of registered first level nurses, working in acute hospital settings, of their changing practice* (pp125–6), the author states that *a qualitative approach was considered most appropriate as it encourages people to reflect at length and in some depth on their experience.*

Given the stated aim of exploring *perceptions*, the choice of a qualitative methodology is clearly quite reasonable as it would be hard to attempt to quantify or measure such perceptions using a methodology from the quantitative paradigm.

Questions posed in quantitative research are about proof, about cause and effect and demonstrating potential associations between **variables**. Quantitative research often starts with a **hypothesis**, which is essentially an idea that is tested using established scientific methods. Hypotheses are often presented as a **null hypothesis** (or the opposite of what the researcher actually expects to find) in order to aid statistical analysis, which will disprove the null hypothesis, or prove the hypothesis, if you like.

Example of a quantitative research hypothesis

In their study of student nurses to compare face-to-face and computer-aided learning (CAL) about hand washing, Bloomfield et al. (2010, p289) posed three null hypotheses:

1. *There would be no difference between the knowledge test scores of nursing students taught the theory of handwashing using CAL when compared with those taught using conventional methods.*
2. *There would be no difference in the handwashing skill performance scores of nursing students taught using CAL when compared with those taught using conventional methods.*
3. *There would be no difference in the retention of handwashing knowledge and skills in nursing students taught handwashing using CAL when compared with those taught by conventional methods.*

These hypotheses appear to reflect the purpose of this form of enquiry, which is to understand whether computer-aided learning can assist the understanding of handwashing over three domains of measurement: knowledge, practice and retention of knowledge.

Qualitative questions seek answers about things that cannot easily be measured or counted. They are more concerned with understanding experiences, opinions and beliefs. Qualitative research starts with a question, an aim or a general statement about something that needs exploring; it does not start with a hypothesis but may be used to generate one.

Example of a qualitative research question

In their ethnographic study on the perception of the risk of falls, Kilian et al. (2008, p331) pose the purpose of their enquiry as being *to examine the perceptions of risk regarding falling held by older adults and their adult children*. Given the **inductive** nature of qualitative research, this aim, which does not contain any reference to what the study might find, appears appropriate to this enquiry.

Critiquing the choice of paradigm, therefore, requires that you know what the two research paradigms are used to investigate and the sorts of questions they can answer. On some occasions it appears evident from the introduction that the answers to the important questions being asked lie in more than one paradigm, and that the researcher may be under-investigating the topic by failing to use a triangulated methodology.

Ethics

Ethics should permeate the whole research process. Good research is ethical research, but sadly not all ethical research is good research. Certainly, it is possible to undertake research that is both ethical and of a high standard, and in many respects producing research ethically adds to the quality of the research process.

When critiquing research from an ethical point of view, there are many questions that can and should be asked. Many students look for some statement that the research has been given ethical clearance, and many regard this as showing that the research is therefore ethically sound. There are two problems with adopting this stance: the first is that not all papers make this statement (Jolley, 2010); and the second is that even with ethical clearance, there may still be questions about the conduct of the research that need to be answered.

Theory

One note of caution for the novice at critiquing is that many journals only accept papers that can demonstrate ethical clearance at the point of submission. In such journals the individual papers will not state that they received ethical clearance. It is worth checking either inside the journal itself or on the journal website where they carry 'information for authors' for a statement about the requirements for demonstrating ethical clearance for all research papers prior to acceptance – not only will this inform your critique but it is likely to impress your marker too.

Critiquing the ethical credentials of a paper starts with asking questions about whether the research was necessary or whether the existing research, which is covered in the background to the paper, suggests it is not. Undertaking research that is unnecessary is ethically questionable because of the use of resources including people's time and energy.

Gaining **consent** is an ethical cornerstone of any research. Gaining true and valid consent is especially challenging in health and social care research because the participants have the potential to be vulnerable. This vulnerability may result from the participants being ill, elderly or in a dependent relationship with the researcher (who may also be their nurse or otherwise involved in their care). Gaining true consent requires the researcher to demonstrate that the participants' agreement to participate has been free from any coercion, either real or potential (Beauchamp and Childress, 2007).

Coupled with the issue of potential coercion are questions about the ability of the individuals to make a choice about whether to take part in a study or not. This freedom of choice is best illustrated in those studies that report that the participants know that they do not have to take part in the study and that they are aware that they can withdraw at any stage without compromising their usual care – although where this is not stated it is hard to know if this principle has been observed.

Consent also requires that the potential participants have the **capacity** (mental ability) to make the choice to participate or not. If there is any doubt about capacity, it is desirable that other sources of consent are sought, for instance from spouses, parents or other guardians (this is sometimes referred to as assent). In studies where there are obvious questions about the capacity of the participants to consent to taking part, it is desirable that the researchers make some statement about ethically managing this.

Example critique: consent

In their observational study of care giving between husband and wife when one has dementia, Jansson et al. (2001, p807) justify gaining consent from people with dementia by stating that *spouses were asked to remind his/her partner about the study every time before the observer's visit*. Given the fact that these people had dementia, there are significant questions about their capacity to consent and therefore about the ethics of the study, although by involving their spouse in the consent process, these researchers can at least be said to have tried all they could to ensure free and informed consent.

Other fundamental questions to be asked of the ethics of a paper include: Do they protect the **confidentiality** and **anonymity** of those involved? Do they appear to have done more good than harm? Did the study answer the question as set and were the resources used in the study used to good effect?

Activity 3.5   *Critical thinking*

Review what your code of conduct says about consent and confidentiality. Reflect on what this means for undertaking nursing research.

Since the links between what the code of conduct says about consent and confidentiality are clear, there is no specimen answer at the end of the chapter.

All of these ethical questions can be asked in the critique, especially where the paper does not explicitly state whether the researchers have addressed them. A good study will not only state what ethical questions there are, but also suggest how these might have been addressed. For example, a good paper will make it clear that the researchers dealt with any upset caused by making counselling and support available.

There are many sources of questions about the ethics of research and how these should apply to the conduct of research in human subjects. Some general ethical principles that guide this questioning have already been identified, but Beauchamp and Childress (2007) identify four important ethical principles that apply to all healthcare practice and might inform a critique. These principles were introduced in Chapter 1 and are: **beneficence** (doing good); **non-maleficence** (avoiding unnecessary harm); **autonomy** (respecting freedom of action) and **justice** (fairness).

Critiquing the ethics of a piece of research is as much about your understanding of what is right, what is wrong and what might be ethically questionable as it is about following a critiquing framework. This is one reason why having an understanding of your code of conduct is important and why you were asked to review it in this chapter.

The discussion and conclusions

The purpose of the discussion and conclusions sections of the paper is to add some context to the results section. Context is achieved by reviewing how well the research has answered the initial question asked (or demonstrated the hypothesis to be true) or not, as well as examining what similar research in the same area has shown and perhaps looking at the policy context within which the findings might operate (Gerish and Lacey, 2006).

The discussion also allows the researcher to explain the results that they have found and why they may have arrived at them. The discussion section of a research paper may be presented in one of two ways: it may be a section on its own or it may be contained within the results section with a discussion attached to each of the results. Either style is reasonable.

From the critiquing point of view, there are two common problems that arise in the discussion sections of published research. First, they may be used to expand on the results rather than explain and contextualise them, and second, the discussion of the results may wander away from a discussion of the questions that were originally posed. This final point can be devastating for a paper that has failed to actually address the question it set out to answer. This wandering of the discussion often points to the use of the wrong methodology or data-collection methods, or to the fact that the authors have been distracted from their main aim by incidental, albeit exciting, findings.

Incidental findings that were not part of the original aim of the research can be of questionable value, as the research design, methodology and methods may not support them. That is to say, the incidental findings may be subject to **biases** that the researcher has not anticipated that may mean the findings are of questionable worth.

Theory

By creating a flow diagram of the contents of a research paper it is easy to identify the initial question or hypothesis that the research set out to answer. This can then be used to compare the results identified in the discussion with the initial aims of the study to see if the two are consistent. Not only does this save time but it adds to the clarity of the process.

The discussion section of the paper is also the place where researchers can discuss the limitations of the study that may arise from practical issues with the implementation of research or from issues that were not fully thought out at the start of the study process. Identifying the methodological and other weaknesses of a study in the discussion and conclusions allows the reader to appreciate some of the tensions that present themselves when trying to do research in the real world.

The best conclusions relate only to the aims of the study and what other research and policy might mean in relation to the findings. It is the nature of nursing and all health and social care research that the findings from a study generate new questions that need answering. Such questions may arise out of the findings of the research, the lack of definitive findings from the research or perhaps contradictions between the study and other previous research or existing policy. The diligent researcher will recognise these issues and will suggest areas for further research, which may be presented as questions or general topic areas.

CHAPTER SUMMARY

This chapter has introduced you to the key elements that need to be considered when setting out to undertake a critique of a piece of research and has established why it is important to be able to critique research before considering applying its findings to nursing practice.

There are many methods available to the novice – and, indeed, to the experienced nurse – that help in the process of appraising a piece of research. These include creating an overview and/or flow diagram of the research to highlight important areas and using a critiquing framework to guide the process.

A variety of issues must be considered when critiquing the title of a research paper, including the credentials of the researchers undertaking the study. Sometimes a degree of detective work is necessary in order to critique these in a meaningful way. All researchers should identify the purpose of the research, and its aims or hypotheses, which will inform the choice of research paradigm and methodology chosen for the study.

Ethical considerations are fundamental to all research. Critiquing requires an appreciation of ethical principles as well as consideration of how these are evidenced within the research process. A good discussion section of a paper should identify what the research has shown in relation to its original aims, as well as how these findings reflect what is already known about the subject and the policy context within which the research might be employed in nursing practice.

Activities: brief outline answers

Activity 3.3: Reflection (page 41)

The first way to quickly ascertain whether a paper is original research is to use the advanced filters that exist in some research engines to ensure that you identify only papers that are empirical research – these are often known as original papers. The second important method is to read the abstract, which will often identify a research aim or question, the methodology used, sampling method applied, data-collection methods used and the key findings, as well as the conclusions of the study.

Activity 3.4: Reflection (page 42)

'Qualitative' tends to suggest notions of quality, and 'quantitative' hints at the fact that something can be counted (think quality and quantity). The philosophical underpinnings of the two approaches lie in the fact that qualitative research is about people's perceptions, understandings and feelings about the world (they are essentially human focused) while quantitative research is concerned with scientific approaches to research that might include understanding cause and effect and counting outcomes.

Knowledge review

Now that you have completed the chapter, how would you rate your knowledge of the following topics?

	Good	Adequate	Poor
1. Why the ability to critique research is important.			
2. The important questions that need to be asked of all research.			
3. Applying a systematic method to the critiquing of research.			

	Good	Adequate	Poor
4. The ethics of the various stages of the research process.			

Where you're not confident in your knowledge of a topic, what will you do next?

Further reading

Ellis, P (2010) *Understanding research for nursing students.* Exeter: Learning Matters.
This book provides a structured introduction to research approaches and methods.

Gerrish, K and Lacey, A (2006) *The research process in nursing* (5th ed.). Oxford: Blackwell.
Chapter 3 on research ethics is an interesting read.

Hek, G and Moule, P (2006) *Making sense of research: an introduction for health and social care practitioners* (3rd ed.). London: Sage.
Chapter 11 on critical appraisal and Appendix 1, a critical appraisal framework, are particularly helpful.

Parahoo, K (2006) *Nursing research: principles, process and issues* (2nd ed.). London: Palgrave Macmillan.
Chapter 17 on critiquing research is very helpful.

Useful websites

www.consort-statement.org/consort-statement/overviewo A structured and helpful website that demonstrates clearly strategies for creating research.
www.eric-on-line.co.uk/index.php The Ethics and Research Information Catalogue contains several interesting articles and web links.
www.nres.npsa.nhs.uk/ This is the home of the National Research Ethics Service for the UK.
www.srs-mcmaster.ca/Default.aspx?tabid=630 This is the McMaster Occupational Therapy Evidence-based Practice group webpage, which has links to qualitative and quantitative research critiquing forms and guidelines.

Chapter 4

Critiquing research: approach-specific elements

Peter Ellis

NMC Standards for Pre-registration Nursing Education (2010)

This chapter will address the following competencies:

Domain 1: Professional values

7. All nurses must be responsible and accountable for keeping their knowledge and skills up to date through continuing professional development. They must aim to improve their performance and enhance the safety and quality of care through evaluation, supervision and appraisal.

9. All nurses must appreciate the value of evidence in practice, be able to understand and appraise research, apply relevant theory and research findings to their work, and identify areas for further investigation.

Essential Skills Clusters

This chapter will address the following ESCs:

Cluster: Care, compassion and communication

1. As partners in the care process, people can trust a newly registered graduate nurse to provide collaborative care based on the highest standards, knowledge and competence.

Cluster: Organisational aspects of care

16. People can trust the newly registered graduate nurse to safely lead, co-ordinate and manage care.

Chapter aims

After reading this chapter, you will be able to:

*   identify the important issues for critique within qualitative research;
*   identify the important issues for critique within quantitative research;
*   demonstrate an understanding of the choices for the different research methods used in qualitative and quantitative research and be able to critique them;
*   describe what good data analysis might look like when critiquing qualitative or quantitative research.

Introduction

The purpose of this chapter is to explore in more depth the critical appraisal processes that are applied when critiquing qualitative or quantitative research. The distinction between the two research approaches (or paradigms) has already been made. This chapter will enable you to decipher what good research practice looks like within each of these paradigms and describe some of the reasons for the practical choices made about methodologies and methods within each approach.

The chapter is split into two sections, the first dealing with qualitative research and the second with quantitative research. It complements the critiquing framework in the appendix to this chapter and together they identify the questions you might ask of research and some of the answers you might expect from a good paper. As in the previous chapter, there are a number of examples of research included within the text. You may find it useful to have some of these to hand when reading this chapter so that you can engage in critical appraisal of them as you read.

It is important that you understand the research process in order to be able to critique it. To this end we strongly suggest that you use at least one, if not more, research textbooks to support your learning and from which to reference your critique.

Critiquing qualitative research

Within this section we will explore the critiquing of qualitative research. Remember, qualitative research asks questions about people's experiences, attitudes, feelings, understandings and opinions. The qualitative paradigm is associated with the social sciences and 'people focused' enquiry; it looks at the world from the point of view of people. On the whole, approaches to qualitative research are inductive, that is, they start from a position of neutrality, ask a question and allow the answer to emerge.

Qualitative research is, therefore, concerned with describing and understanding human experiences as they occur and are interpreted in real life. In critiquing qualitative research attention focuses on the **credibility** of the evidence presented as an authentic account and accurate interpretation of the respondents' viewpoints in relation to the research questions being explored.

The choice of methodology

We identified in Chapter 3 that the research paradigm upon which a research paper is based has to do with the school of thought upon which it is based. Methodologies are a more detailed plan of action used to undertake the research – the road map, if you like. Within qualitative research the different methodologies provide a structure for undertaking the research and are selected because of how well they actually fit the question asked.

Example critique: choice of methodology

In their study of adaptation to life after acquired brain injury (ABI), Parsons and Stanley (2008, p232) state that they chose **phenomenology** as their methodology because they were seeking to gain an in-depth insight into the *lived experience of people with ABI*. This aligns well with the express purpose of phenomenological research, which is to explore the lived experience of participants (Ellis, 2010).

Example critique continued

> However, as this study engaged only two participants it would be reasonable to suggest that they might equally well have used a **case study** or **biographic** methodology while accepting that phenomenology is also a perfectly acceptable choice.

Many qualitative research papers do not identify a specific research methodology – they are called **generic** or **exploratory qualitative studies**. This is not, usually, a mistake on the part of the researchers; rather, it is a practical response to the fact that the question they are asking does not fit neatly into one of the established methodologies. In a critique it is often sufficient to point this out and perhaps suggest a methodology that might have been chosen or, alternatively, a means of adjusting the question to make it potentially fit a particular approach.

Table 4.1 shows the main research methodologies used in qualitative research and gives some idea of the type of issues they are used to study.

Research methodologies are, therefore, the overall scheme by which research is undertaken, and the choice of methodology is driven by the exact research question being asked. For example, a question about what it is like to work on a cancer ward suggests the use of **ethnography**, while developing a theory about how people cope with life with cancer will suggest that the study methodology should be **grounded theory**.

When critiquing the choice of methodology chosen for a piece of research it is worth looking at the sometimes subtle differences between the methodologies and perhaps suggesting, rather than categorically stating, how a slightly modified question might have led the researchers to have used a different methodology. Where the methodology chosen appears to fit well with the question being asked, it is important to state why this is the case as in the example critique earlier.

Sampling

When critiquing the choice of sampling methods and sample size in qualitative research it is worth remembering what qualitative research seeks to do. Qualitative research seeks to inform the thinking about a topic and seeks for its findings to be potentially **transferable** to other similar situations. This means that the findings are not said to be directly applicable – generalisable – to other similar situations, but they might inform decision making – especially where the findings are supported by other, similar research.

In biographic and case study research, the sample may be as few as one individual rising up to dozens in ethnographic research. Most qualitative research methodologies,

Table 4.1: Potential areas for study and their associated qualitative methodologies

Methodology	What it studies
Ethnography	Studies cultures and groups and how they interact
Grounded theory	Generates, or develops a theory about a social interaction
Phenomenology	Describes the **essence** or perceived reality of an experience
Case study research	Explores case(s) of interest
Generic qualitative	Studies people's attitudes, beliefs, opinions or experiences

for example phenomenological or grounded theory research, use sample sizes of between six and 15 participants.

There are a number of characteristics of qualitative sampling that relate it to the purpose of the topic being studied. Since most qualitative research is about understanding individuals' perceptions and experiences, sampling involves identifying individuals who have had the experience that is being studied. Selecting people because of their common experience is called **purposive sampling** (Streubert Speziale and Carpenter, 2007). Because the individuals within the sample are similar on account of the shared experience, the sample may also be said to be **homogeneous**. In qualitative research this is seen as a good feature of the research design, so long as the people selected represent the sorts of people that the research question is about.

Homogeneous and purposive sampling means that the findings of qualitative research may be transferable to other similar people in similar situations and context – **transferability**. A note of caution however, while the sample is said to be homogeneous due to a commonality of experience it is not necessarily so in terms of the interpretation of the experience as reality is said to be experienced in multiple ways in qualitative research.

Concept summary: purposive sampling

Purposive sampling refers to the fact that individuals are selected because they fit the purpose of the study – their purpose is to be able to talk about whatever phenomenon is being studied. Individuals within such samples are also similar in that they share an experience or some other feature(s) in common; this is referred to as homogeneity, which literally means being the same – at least in respect of one important variable. However, this does not mean that they view the experience in the same way necessarily. When critiquing qualitative samples it is desirable that the characteristics of the individuals in a sample are identified to the reader and that you can understand who has been selected for the study and why. Understanding the characteristics and context of the research aids the reader in understanding how transferable the findings of the study might be to the place that they work and the people that they work with.

Many qualitative studies select participants from groups of individuals who are easily identified and handy to approach. These **convenience samples**, as they are called, are an acceptable way of recruiting participants to study (Parahoo, 2006). When such samples contain individuals who may be vulnerable, it is good practice to show within the sampling how this has been accounted for. Strategies may include approaching the individuals through a third party (such as another member of staff that they know, or a relative or friend).

Example critique: purposive and convenience sampling

In their study of the lived experiences of diabetes among elderly, rural-dwelling people, George and Thomas (2010, p1094) used a *purposive sample . . . drawn from local agencies on ageing . . . English speaking people aged 65–85 years . . . all confined to their homes and living in a rural area. . . . with diabetes.* It is clear from

Example critique: continued

their description that all of the participants were selected to suit the purposes of the research *to elucidate experiences and perceptions of self-management of their diabetes as narrated by older people with insulin-dependent diabetes living in a rural area* (George and Thomas, 2010, p1094). Evidently, the sample included only English-speaking people and those willing to discuss their disease; this will limit the transferability of the findings, but it is a reasonable practical way of sampling in qualitative research. The identification of people via local agencies that care for the elderly demonstrates that this is a convenience sample. Being a convenience sample raises some questions about whether the participants felt coerced in to participating in order to please the care agencies.

Activity 4.1	*Reflection*

Reflect on how you respond to approaches for help or information from different people. What factors influence the responses that you give and in what situations do you feel more obliged to comply with the request? How might this reflect in the ways in which people respond to requests to become involved in research in the hospital or other clinical setting?

There are some possible answers at the end of the chapter.

Many qualitative studies use the point of **data saturation** as an idealised way of determining the size of the sample to be studied. Data from the interview or focus groups are analysed as the study progresses, and recruitment stops when no new ideas are emerging from the data – that is, when the data is **saturated** (Macnee and McCabe, 2008). This is a very reasonable approach to use in qualitative research and may be positively critiqued.

One other common approach to sampling, which is frequently used in grounded theory, is called **theoretical sampling** (Glaser and Strauss, 1967). Theoretical sampling occurs when the researcher has analysed early interviews within the study and has started to create some initial theories. This analysis leads the researcher to ask additional questions and prompts them to purposively recruit further participants to the study who are suitable to help answer emerging questions or to firm up the emerging theory. This is an extension of the idea of data saturation and makes good sense within qualitative methodologies.

The best qualitative research papers will therefore identify the characteristics of their sample, the recruitment and sampling method used as well as demonstrating how they have tried to go about this process in an ethical manner.

The choice of data-collection methods

Methods refer to the tools used to collect the data for a research project. When critiquing data-collection methods within qualitative research, it is important, as ever, to bear in mind: the purpose of the research (which arises from the research question), the chosen methodology, and the capabilities and vulnerabilities of the people being researched. The nature of the research question will strongly determine the sense of the data-collection method being used.

Within qualitative research there are four main approaches to data-collection: interviews, focus groups, observation and examination of artefacts. Certainly, the choice of the data-collection method will relate strongly not only to the topic under investigation but also to the characteristics of the participants.

For example, it might be reasonable to question a qualitative study that enquired into the nature of some potentially embarrassing topic (such as sexually transmitted diseases) using a focus group. It is clearly more appropriate (regardless of the methodology) to ask such questions in a one-to-one interview.

Example critique: data collection using focus groups

In their study of young children's understanding of mental health, Roose and John (2003) used focus groups to discover children's understanding of mental health and the availability of services for mental health services among their age group. On face value this seems like a potentially difficult format for data collection given the emotive nature of mental health problems. Roose and John (2003, p546) fail to justify their choice of method, merely stating that *focus groups were identified as the most appropriate way to explore younger children's views of services and their understanding of mental health*. They do, however, seem to have thought about the potential effects of the focus group by asking the school teachers to identify students with no mental health problems who were likely to be interested in the topic and would be comfortable in a group. Despite their careful selection, it would be reasonable to ask if one-to-one interviews might not have been more appropriate given the nature of the topic and the possibility of covert power relationships within the groups.

Where there are potential power relationships, or when individuals may be vulnerable in other ways, it may not be appropriate to use focus groups or observations to collect qualitative data. In these instances the usefulness of the chosen methods has to take second place to the ethical principles of avoiding harm and respecting autonomy.

Activity 4.2 *Critical thinking*

In what sorts of situations might you feel less able to speak your mind than others? Why is this and why might this answer help you to understand how research participants view data-collection methods in qualitative research?

There are some possible answers at the end of the chapter.

Observational data collection may be a benefit in studies that seek to find out what people do or how they behave in certain situation. The use of observation may not be the correct method when the purpose of the study is to understand an issue from the perspective of the participant. Observation just does not fit the purpose – it is used to see what people do rather than study what they think. Observation followed by interviews or a focus group discussion, however, may be an appropriate choice of method when the research is seeking to understand what people do and why in a particular situation.

In some research methodologies, for example ethnography, there is a clear need for the use of multiple methods of data collection. Ethnography seeks to understand the culture and behaviours within a group; this requires a mix of observation, participation in the group and interviews (Parahoo, 2006). Some ethnography may also include the examination of artefacts such as pictures and letters in an effort to understand their meaning to the group. Failure to undertake at least two levels of data collection within ethnography would give cause for concern and raise questions about the completeness of the data collection.

Some questions around data collection in the qualitative methodologies are somewhat more subtle. For example, there remain questions about the use of semi-structured interviews in phenomenology where the consensus view used to be that the interviews should be unstructured. In many critical appraisals it would be reasonable to point this out without committing to one argument or the other.

Critiquing qualitative research methods, therefore, requires the reviewer to make some judgement about the justification that the researcher has made for their choice of methods. It also requires the reviewer to ask questions of themselves about what approach they would use when trying to obtain the same sorts of information from people in similar circumstances.

The analysis and results

The data that are produced in qualitative research are words. These words need sorting, grouping and interpreting in order to help make sense of the data collected for a study. There are several stages that can add **credibility** and **rigour** to this process and demonstrate the researcher's commitment to producing research findings that are transparent and high quality.

Concept summary: credibility

Credibility refers to how believable a piece of qualitative research is. The use of the term in relation to qualitative research suggests that the research undertaken actually answers what it set out to answer because of the quality of the way in which the research has been done.

Rigour in qualitative research suggests that the research process has been undertaken in a well-thought-through, fully explained and transparent manner. It also requires that this is fully explained to those reading the paper.

There is no single right way in which to examine qualitative data. What is always important in the qualitative data analysis is that the process is well explained and that the decisions made in the process appear logical and transparent (credible and rigorous). This transparency requires that the paper explains exactly how the data were analysed and by whom, and what strategies they put in place to confirm the conclusions that they came to.

It should be apparent that the study has been conducted in a neutral manner and that the findings have been allowed to emerge – that is, the whole research process has been inductive and not based on confirming a pre-existing hypothesis. This neutrality of the data analysis process is said to bring **confirmability** to the study (Polit and Beck, 2008).

Commonly, papers will say that the author(s) read and reread the data (usually **verbatim** transcripts of interviews or focus groups) looking for common ideas and themes identifying the issues that were most important to the participants. This is a reasonable approach to data analysis, although many qualitative researchers are now using computer programs. What is important in critiquing the analysis of qualitative research is not so much the strategy used but the supplementary strategies used to check the credibility and trustworthiness of this initial data analysis approach.

Key among the strategies used to confirm the findings of a study are the use of a second person to review the data collected – be they transcripts of interviews or focus groups, video or notes from observations of other artefacts – and come to their own conclusions about the findings. There may be some discussion about how a consensus view about the study results was then arrived at.

The best studies using a single method (such as interviews or focus groups) will further check, and report on, the credibility of their findings in one of two ways. The first is to return the results to some, if not all, of the participants asking the question 'Is this interpretation of the interview a good representation of what you said?' The second approach is to present the findings to other researchers, or people with a special knowledge of the area of investigation, who are encouraged to ask probing questions about the methods used and the findings arrived at (Polit and Beck, 2006).

In studies employing more than one data-collection method the consistency of the findings between the different data-collection methods may be used to demonstrate the degree of credibility of the research. Where more than one data collector is used or different approaches employed, the study should demonstrate a consistency in the data collection; this is termed **dependability**.

A further strategy that helps the reader understand and perhaps come to some agreement with the findings of qualitative research is the use of verbatim (that is, word-for-word) quotes from the participants of the research alongside the themes and categories identified by the researcher. This allows the reader to understand how they have arrived at the findings that they have and to develop an awareness of why the researchers have come to the conclusions that they have. Clearly, the interpretation of what a research participant has said relies to some extent on the context of the conversation in which they said it; nevertheless, verbatim quotes give the critical reviewer a view into the world of the research participant that is missing in studies that do not use them.

Example critique: establishing credibility

In his study of adolescents coping with mood disorder, Meadus (2007) used peer debriefing by two specialist nurses to improve the credibility of the study. He justifies not using the participants to validate his findings by referring to some researchers who say that member checks are not useful in validating results; however, he does not explain whyshe accepts this view. Meadus does provide verbatim quotes from the participants to allow the reader the opportunity to decide if they agree with his interpretation.

While the findings of qualitative research are not said to be generalisable (necessarily applicable) to other people similar to the participants, the existence in the discussion of other similar research showing similar findings demonstrates that the study has some transferability to other groups of individuals.

Critiquing quantitative research

Quantitative research is research that uses numbers and statistics; it is concerned with cause and effect, exposures and outcomes. Key among the concerns for quantitative research are that it should be **valid**, **reliable** and generalisable.

> *Concept summary: validity, reliability and generalisability*
>
> Validity is the ability of a data-collecting tool (a method) to measure what it is supposed to be measuring. For example, we know that a sphygmomanometer (when used properly) will measure blood pressure; however, it is much more difficult to know how well a questionnaire designed to measure anxiety levels actually does so because it may be hard to define what anxiety is. In many studies of anxiety and stress the data collected from questionnaires are supplemented by taking biological samples and measuring the level of cortisol (a hormone associated with stress) in them, as a way of validating the findings.
>
> Reliability refers to the reproducibility of the results of the study. Reliability may refer to whether the data-collection tool (such as a questionnaire) produces broadly similar results when used again in the same population, when applied to the same sample at a different time or when the tool is used by another researcher.
>
> Generalisability refers to the extent to which the findings from a piece of research can be extended out to the general population of people in a similar position – that is, whether the sample used in the research is representative enough of the population to which the findings of the research are to be applied.

Many quantitative studies focus on answering a question which is posed as a hypothesis, which we described earlier as being an idea that is tested using the scientific method. By their nature quantitative studies are therefore **deductive**, setting out to answer the question of the research using a method best suited to establishing the truth, or otherwise, of the initial hypothesis.

The choice of methodology

As with all research, the methodology (which is the broad plan of action for the study) has to fit the questions being asked. The wrong choice of methodology means that a study cannot answer the questions it set out to answer. When critiquing the choice of methodology it is important to understand what each of the different methodologies can be used to research. For example, cause and effect can only be examined with any confidence in experimental studies (which include randomised controlled trials) and cohort studies as these are **prospective** and **longitudinal** (that is, they collect data as things happen over a period of time). Quantitative methods that are not both prospective and longitudinal cannot make this claim as they do not collect data in a forward-going real-time manner.

Table 4.2 shows the sorts of questions that the various quantitative methodologies can be used to answer.

While Table 4.2 is not an exhaustive list of the quantitative methodologies, it provides some clarity as to what the different methods can do. In terms of critiquing the choice of quantitative research methodologies, perhaps the most important question is whether the chosen approach is suitable for examining cause-and-effect relationships.

This is perhaps best understood by remembering that all quantitative methodologies are concerned with the quality of the measurement of variables, where variables are any

Table 4.2: Questions that different quantitative methodologies can be used to answer

Questions	Methodology
If x is done, what will happen? If x is done, how often will y happen?	Experiment/quasi-experiment/ randomised controlled trial.
If a person is exposed to x, will they develop outcome (disease) x? Does exposure to x cause outcome y?	Cohort studies.
What exposure x might have caused this individual to have outcome y?	Case-control studies.
In this group of people how many have been exposed to x or have outcome y? What is the prevalence of x or y in this group?	Cross-sectional studies.
The data show that when x increases in the population so too does y. Might they be associated? When exposure x increases and outcome y increases is there potential that the two are associated in some way?	Ecological studies.

Source: Ellis, 2010.

factors within a study that may differ (vary) between study participants. The quality of the measurements, and therefore the validity and reliability of the study, relies heavily on the elimination of bias within the research process.

Concept summary: bias

Bias is defined as a deviation from the truth. Bias occurs when a deviation from the truth is the result of defects in the way in which a study is carried out. For example, **recall bias** occurs where a study relies on the memory of participants, for example remembering what they ate last week, recalling their alcohol intake over a period of time or whether or not they have ever had chickenpox.

Because, in the examples given, these variables are not being measured in real time (prospectively) or over a period of time (longitudinally) or, indeed, in a standardised way (which will affect both validity and reliability), there is a degree of uncertainty about how good the quality of the data collected actually is.

Taking these issues into account identifies why studies that seek to prove cause and effect need to be prospective and longitudinal, while those that seek only to measure the amount of a certain variable or demonstrate an association or correlation (which conceptually are not as strong as demonstrating cause-and-effect relationships) do not.

Example critique: choice of methodology

Williams et al. (2009) set out to investigate – using a validated personality assessment questionnaire – personality differences specifically related to caring between a group of female staff nurses and a group of female controls. They chose a case-control study as they wanted to look at the differences in personality but were not trying to show a cause-and-effect relationship – merely an association.

This is a reasonable choice of methodology: it would not be possible to show that a more caring disposition creates the desire to be a nurse as the study did not take place before the staff nurses joined the nursing profession and it may be that being a nurse has made the nurse more caring than their non-nursing peers.

When critiquing the choice of methodology, therefore, it is important to identify the expressed purpose of the study and the level of proof associated with it. Identifying the purpose of the study will indicate whether the methodology needs to be prospective and longitudinal or not.

Activity 4.3	Critical thinking

Consider the strict criteria applied to proof in quantitative research – validity requires that what is supposed to be measured is measured and reliability requires that what is measured is done in a consistent manner. Now spend a few minutes writing down everything that you ate and drank exactly one week ago. Now write down everything that you have eaten or drunk today. Which one do you have the most faith in and why?

There are some possible answers and thoughts at the end of the chapter.

Sampling

When thinking about the quality of the sampling methods applied in quantitative research, it is important to remember that the key purpose of this form of enquiry is to produce data that are generalisable. That is to say, quantitative studies seek to produce results that can be applied beyond the sample in which the study took place. To be generalisable, therefore, quantitative studies need to have samples that are **representative** of people who are broadly similar to all the people whom the study is about.

Concept summary: representativeness

Representativeness is about the degree to which the study sample is comparable to the population from which it was taken (for example, in relation to gender, age, ethnicity and severity of disease). The more typical the sample is with regard to the population the study is about, the more likely the findings of the study hold true in that population (generalisability).

In terms of critiquing, this means that the sample used for the study should represent the sorts of people who are identified in the study question. For example, a study of the understanding of dietary management among people newly diagnosed with diabetes should identify what it means by diabetes (type 1 or type 2) as well as what it means by newly diagnosed (say, in the last six months). The selection of potential participants for the study would then be focused on all people who fit these criteria; this would be termed the **study population**.

In some research, all the people in this population might be studied, especially when the population is drawn from a small geographic area or from people with a rare disease – that is, assuming they all consented to participate. Studies that employ this type of sample might include **cross-sectional studies**.

In more sophisticated studies, such as experimental studies, the selection of people from a large potential study population allows everyone the same chance of being included in the study. This is called **probability sampling** and produces a **study sample**. If the sample size is large enough (as calculated using statistical formulae), it can produce a sample that is representative of the larger population – and hence generalisable results.

Where a paper does not identify the processes that occurred in relation to forming the study sample, there are questions that need to be asked about the quality of the sampling, the potential for the introduction of bias and therefore about how generalisable the findings of such research can be.

Activity 4.4   *Critical thinking*

Consider what you have learnt about generalisability and try to identify why this might be an important feature of quantitative research.

There is a possible answer at the end of the chapter.

In **randomised controlled trials** (RCTs) the process goes a step further. Because RCTs seek to examine the difference in outcomes between two or more similar groups to investigate the effectiveness of an intervention, there is a need for the two groups to be broadly similar at the start of the study. So in an RCT you would expect to see that the study sample is further divided into cases (participants to whom the intervention/study drug is given) and controls (participants to who get a dummy intervention or drug). This process must happen randomly (to avoid introducing **selection bias** to the study) and all good RCTs will identify how this is achieved.

Example critique: randomised sample

In their study of the use of the essential oil Lavandin to reduce pre-operative stress, Braden, Reichow and Halm (2009) selected a convenience sample of patients presenting for surgery in one hospital. They included English-speaking patients over 18 who were capable of consenting and were not allergic to Lavandin.
Braden et al. (2009, p350) state that:

Patients were then randomly assigned to one of three groups: (1) Control group that received standard preoperative care, which may include

Example critique continued

> *therapeutic communication, family involvement at the bedside, and pharmacological agents to reduce anxiety; (2) lavandin experimental group, which, in addition to receiving standard care, received essential oils before surgery; and (3) jojoba sham group, which also received standard care as well as a placebo.*
>
> Randomisation was achieved by way of a card system (the researcher drew a card to decide which group the participant was allocated to), although it is not clear what this means exactly. Nor is it clear if, because of the nature of the sample selected, the findings of the study are generalisable to the whole population, although it may well apply to all the sorts of patients attending that particular hospital for elective surgery

In some cases where the splitting of the groups cannot happen randomly, there remain questions about the quality of the research process, especially around the introduction of bias. While it would be correct to critique this element of the research, allowances have to be made where the decision not to create the groups randomly was a practical consideration – for example, when it is hard to hide from the participants and the researchers which group the individual participant has been allocated to.

In case-control studies the selection of cases is based on them having the outcome (usually a disease) of interest with controls being similar in as many other respects as possible (for example, age, gender, ethnicity, income group and educational attainment). In matched cohort studies the controls are chosen because they are similar to the cases being studied in as many respects as possible other than being exposed to the potential cause of the disease under study. In both types of study it is the role of the researcher to create a convincing argument as to why they chose the control groups they did, and the best papers will identify the limitations of the study that arise from the compromises made in this process somewhere in the discussion.

Many quantitative papers identify a starting sample but appear to report data from a smaller sample in the results. This is usually the result of losses to the study from people withdrawing for any number of reasons. It is reasonable to criticise a study in which this occurs when the reasons for, and the characteristics of, the withdrawals are not discussed. There are good reasons for this.

Some withdrawals may be related to some aspect of the thing being studied, for example, a side effect of a drug. Significant numbers of withdrawals from a study because of a side effect may not have statistical, but may have important clinical, implications. Withdrawal of certain groups of people from the study, perhaps older patients or those of a particular gender, may mean that the findings of the study are skewed and that they can no longer claim to be generalisable. Clearly, in a study of two arms such as an RCT, significant withdrawals from the treatment arm may mean that the new drug or intervention is unacceptable to many people and may not be as clinically successful as the researchers suggest. This is worthy of an unambiguous negative critique.

The choice of data-collection methods

We have already made the assertion that all quantitative methodologies are concerned with the quality of the measurement of variables. Nowhere within the quantitative research process is this more obvious than in the choice of data-collection methods. Essentially, there are two elements to data-collection methods that are open to potential critique. The first is the actual choice of the tool itself and its potential to be able to measure whatever it is that it is trying to measure – its validity. Second is the issue of how the tool is actually put to work, how reliable the way in which it was used is.

The most frequently used data-collection tools used in nursing research are questionnaires and other forms of surveys. In many cases the variables that a study seeks to measure are already the subjects of well-tried and tested questionnaires, the validity of which is well established. The best research papers will identify why they chose the questionnaire(s) and how well these might apply to the people they are studying. Poorer quality papers will identify what tools they used but give little or no explanation as to why.

Activity 4.5	*Research and finding out*

There are a large number of questionnaires that exist to measure diverse health and socially related variables in research. These tools can be used to measure variables such as quality of life, mental well-being and levels of anxiety either generally or in relation to specific diseases. Go online and try to identify some of these and read about what it is they are designed to be able to measure. You may find this useful to do when critiquing a paper.

There are some websites identified at the end of this chapter where you could go to look at some questionnaires.

Other data for quantitative studies may be collected from existing sources such as databases and medical and nursing records. The quality of this data will vary greatly and the best studies will make allowances for this and may make some efforts to check the quality of both the data and the accuracy and consistency (reliability) of the collection of it for research purposes (especially where more than one person is used for data collection).

Physiological and biological data are frequently collected in quantitative studies. The quality of these forms of data is thought by many nurses to be beyond question; this is not, however, always the case. For example, blood pressure measurements, even when undertaken using the same apparatus, vary between individuals. The best quality research will try to minimise this difference by training all those involved to use the same method to take blood pressures and thereby increase reliability.

With regard to biological and physiological data, the best papers will record how specimens and measurements were taken, by whom, under what conditions, where, how often and how data-collection staff were trained. In some of the best research reports there will be data on the degree of agreement between different data-collection staff, typically measured in statistical terms.

The analysis and results

The analysis of quantitative research invariably requires the use of statistics. These statistics are of two separate kinds. The first are **descriptive statistics**, the purpose of which is to describe the study sample and perhaps some of the outcomes. The best research papers will contain descriptive statistics that explain the frequency, spread and measures of central tendency (for example, the **means** and **medians**) of the data.

Such data should give you a good idea of some of the characteristics of the study participants, such as their ages and gender. In comparison studies such as RCTs and matched cohorts, the reader should also be able to see that the two groups are broadly similar in all described variables at the start of the study – if they appear not to be so, this would give cause for critique.

The second form of statistics used are what are referred to as **inferential statistics**. These statistics described the levels of confidence that the researchers place in their findings and are derived from applying various statistical tests.

There are a large number of statistical tests that can be applied to numerical data, and the best papers leave the reader in no doubt about what tests have been used and which statistical packages. Clearly, it is beyond the scope of this text to delve into these now; however, there are many good guides that explain which statistical tests apply to which forms of data and in what circumstances.

Activity 4.6 *Research and finding out*

There are a large number of statistical tests that can be applied to numerical data. Go online and try to identify some of these and read about what it is they are designed to do. You may find this strategy useful when critiquing a paper.

There are some websites identified at the end of this chapter where you could look at examples of statistics used with different forms of data.

The analysis and presentation of results within quantitative research can be quite confusing because of the numbers involved. The best papers will, however, present their findings in a variety of ways including graphs, tables and charts, many of which are fairly simple to understand and interpret. It is not a matter for critique that the reader is not familiar with the approach to analysis employed. A good critique will involve the novice reader in learning some things about the basic elements of what they are reading and applying it.

C H A P T E R   S U M M A R Y

The approach to critiquing either form of research is driven by what the research ultimately aims to do. The choice of research methodology, and whether or not it is qualitative or quantitative, should have been informed by the exact questions, the nature of those questions and the type of person about whom the research seeks to find answers.

There are various approaches to identifying and recruiting samples for both qualitative and quantitative research, and these are driven by both theoretical and practical issues. Similarly, there are a number of different methods that can be used to collect data, and it is the role of the researcher to defend the choices they made.

As with all stages of the research process, the choice of data-collection method arises out of both theoretical and practical considerations. Researchers need to make it plain why they make the choices they do. While recognising this, a good critique may include some suggestions about why the method might or might not be the best choice, as well as suggestions for other methods of data collection.

The analysis of data is a process that needs justification in the qualitative paradigm, and explanation and transparency in both qualitative and quantitative research.

Activities: brief outline answers

Activity 4.1: Reflection (page 54)

The ways in which we are approached and by whom certainly have an effect on the ways in which we respond to requests for help. We feel obligations to people that employ us, people that we work with and our family. These obligations arise from a sense of duty, belonging and, in the case of family, love, and may conflict with our own true wishes. Approaches in person are harder to ignore, while those in writing or via e-mail may prove easier to ignore.

Asking people who are patients to become involved in research may create dilemmas for them where they, too, feel a sense of obligation arising out of duty to respond to the care they have received, the desire to belong and please their carers and perhaps affection and gratitude. As suggested in the text, this may mean that researchers have to explore ways for patient participants to exercise freedom of choice in relation to research, which may mean making it easy to say no or simply ignore a written request.

Activity 4.2: Critical thinking (page 55)

There are often potential issues within qualitative research that need to be accounted for in the choice of data-collection methods. These include power relationships between the researcher and the participant – and, indeed, between participants themselves. For instance, you may not feel able to talk openly about how you feel about your job in front of your boss and you may not want to talk about your home life in front of your colleagues.

Similarly, participants in research are not likely to want to discuss certain issues in a focus group format, and if they do, they may choose not to be completely truthful, so the choice of method will impact on the credibility of the research findings.

Activity 4.3: Critical thinking (page 60)

It is likely that you can remember virtually everything that you ate and drank today, while your memory of what you ate and drank even as little as a week ago is a little vague. Contemporary collection of data, which would require that you kept a food and drink diary as you ate and drank, would be more accurate as there is little room for error. Depending on the degree of accuracy needed you might even choose to weigh or measure what you eat and drink. This demonstrates that prospective data collection allows for accuracy and eliminates the need for recall (known as recall bias).

Why then longitudinal? Clearly, if you want to know if diet is associated with disease, then a one-off measure of diet is no good. To ensure accuracy of data collection you would want prospective food diaries kept over a period of time (prospectively). Gathering data prospectively also allows the collection of data on other things that might be causes that might be associated with the outcome (disease) that you are interested in, such as smoking, exercise or occupation.

Activity 4.4: Critical thinking (page 61)

Quantitative research seeks to provide answers to many clinical problems. It is important, therefore, that the approaches to solving these problems are ones that can be used with confidence in all similar clinical situations. For example, it is important to know that a particular tablet will reduce blood pressure or that a dressing regime will improve the healing of a wound.

Knowledge review

Now that you have completed the chapter, how would you rate your knowledge of the following topics?

	Good	Adequate	Poor
1. Methods for demonstrating research quality in qualitative research.			
2. Methods for demonstrating research quality in quantitative research.			
3. The pros and cons of some data-collection methods in qualitative and quantitative research.			
4. The elements that go into good data analysis in qualitative and quantitative research.			

Where you're not confident in your knowledge of a topic, what will you do next?

Further reading

Coughlan, M, Cronin, P and Ryan, F (2007) Step-by-step guide to critiquing research. Part 1: quantitative research. *British Journal of Nursing*, 16 (11): 658–63.
This is a reasonable overview of critiquing quantitative research.

Ellis, P (2010) *Understanding research for nursing students.* Exeter: Learning Matters.
A student's guide to research.

Hek, G and Moule, P (2006) *Making sense of research: an introduction for health and social care practitioners* (3rd ed.). London: Sage.
Chapter 11 on critical appraisal and Appendix 1, a critical appraisal framework, are particularly helpful.

Parahoo, K (2006) *Nursing research: principles, process and issues* (2nd ed.). London: Palgrave Macmillan.
Chapter 17 on critiquing research is very helpful.

Ryan, F, Coughlan, M and Cronin, P (2007) Step-by-step guide to critiquing research. Part 2: qualitative research, *British Journal of Nursing*, 16 (12): 738–44.
This is a reasonable overview of critiquing qualitative research.

Silverman, D (2004) *Doing qualitative research: a practical handbook.* London: Sage.
A good guide to undertaking qualitative research.

Useful websites

http://statpages.org/ A very useful statistics resource.
www.graphpad.com/www/book/choose.htm Contains a useful table giving an overview of statistical tests.

www.srs-mcmaster.ca/Default.aspx?tabid=630 The McMaster Occupational Therapy Evidence-based Practice group web page, which has links to qualitative and quantitative research critiquing forms and guidelines.

Websites containing validated data-collection questionnaires

www.healthmeasurement.org/Measures.html A website with links to and descriptions of a number of widely used validated questionnaires.

www.sf-36.org/ Short form 36 is widely to use to measure self-reported quality of life and functionality.

Chapter 5

Making sense of subjective experience

Lioba Howatson-Jones

NMC Standards for Pre-registration Nursing Education (2010)

This chapter will address the following competencies:

Domain 1: Professional values

9. All nurses must appreciate the value of evidence in practice, be able to understand and appraise research, apply relevant theory and research findings to their work, and identify areas for further investigation.

Domain 3: Nursing practice and decision-making

1. All nurses must use up-to-date knowledge and evidence to assess, plan, deliver and evaluate care, communicate findings, influence change and promote health and best practice. They must make person-centred, evidence-based judgments and decisions, in partnership with others involved in the care process, to ensure high quality care.

Essential Skills Clusters

This chapter will address the following ESCs:

Cluster: Care, compassion and communication

3. People can trust the newly registered graduate nurse to respect them as individuals and strive to help them to preserve their dignity at all times.

Chapter aims

After reading this chapter, you will be able to:

- identify how subjective experience relates to other forms of evidence;
- understand the role of subjective experience in the interpretation of evidence;
- discuss particular stances that might be adopted;
- contextualise lived experience.

Introduction

This chapter explains how subjective experience needs to be considered alongside objective and more rational forms of evidence. It will help you to start to make sense of your experience and identify how this might fit with other forms of evidence. The chapter addresses questions of why it might be that in an era of scientific certainty and effectiveness, professionals feel increasingly anxious and uncertain about the delivery of care and patients feel increasingly uncared for. It is important that healthcare does not become objectified as 'something' we do to others as opposed to recognising it as something we do with 'someone' and that a range of evidence is utilised to support practice, as appropriate.

The chapter begins by exploring subjective experience from the perspective of the nurse as well as that of the patient. This experience is then related to other forms of evidence such as objective data, research findings and audit. The role that subjectivity still plays in the interpretation and implementation of rational knowledge is considered further and related to the stances that may be adopted. The chapter closes by contextualising the lived experience of practitioners in relation to making sense of the multiple dimensions of the evidence base of their practice.

Subjective experience

Subjective experience can be defined as how we make sense of a situation, how it affects us individually and what we feel about it. We learn from the experiences we have because through interaction with our physical and social environment, we develop knowledge (this notion of experiential evidence is reflected in Figure 1.1 in Chapter 1 (page 16) as one of the influences on practice). This knowledge may be modified as we encounter and respond to different situations. Such knowledge may be consciously considered when thinking cognitively and reflectively about what is taking place. However, sometimes we are not aware of the learning taken from experiences until it emerges as intuitive knowing.

Intuitive knowledge is difficult to articulate precisely because there is a lack of awareness of its existence – only that the nurse seems to 'sense' what to do in practice. Subjective experience and subjective knowledge are influenced, in part, by our histories as well as cultural understanding.

Benner's (1984) study of the development and progression of nursing knowledge identified intuitive knowing as an essential part of the advancing practice of the experienced nurse. This means that in complex situations the experienced nurse is able to identify solutions to problems that are difficult to explain but that they know to be right, for example, dealing with emergencies or recognising unusual features within routine practice. Intuition and empathy form a part of such experiential knowing that is not easily rationalised, more tentative and, therefore, uncertain (Heron, 1996). Such abstractions have been called 'sixth sense, instinct and gut feeling' (Muir, 2004, p50). Benner's (1984) work and that of Muir (2004) are founded on the principle that intuition resulting from experience provides a substantial evidence base for practice. This contrasts with more analytical approaches that consider the evidence surrounding experience and actions taken in order to substantiate the knowledge used. Consider the following case study to identify how this might work in practice.

CASE STUDY: Detecting a case of tracheal stricture

Anja had been involved in a motorcycle accident while on holiday in Cyprus, where she had sustained extensive head injuries. These had left her in a **vegetative state**, although she was able to breathe on her own through a **tracheostomy tube** with supplementary oxygen. Anja had been transferred back to a hospital in the UK for assessment and the planning of her ongoing care. She was not suitable for admission to an intensive care unit or a high-dependency ward as her condition was categorised as chronic rather than acute, but Anja still required special nursing, particularly at night. Consequently, a number of flexi nurses were drafted in to help with her care.

During a night shift Maureen – the nurse on duty – noticed that Anja seemed restless and 'just did not look right'. Anja's **vital signs** and **pulse oximetry** that Maureen recorded were within normal parameters for Anja, and there was no apparent incontinence or reason for discomfort as she was nursed on an airflow pressure mattress. Maureen decided to check the tracheostomy tube, first undertaking tracheal suction and then changing the tube, even though the pulse oximeter reading was normal. Anja remained restless.

Maureen was still not happy with Anja's condition although she could not account for this. Maureen asked the anaesthetist to come and review Anja. The anaesthetist, who was relatively inexperienced, examined Anja and could also not find anything specific but called other medical colleagues for their opinion. By this stage an hour had elapsed and Maureen noticed a sudden significant drop in Anja's oximetry reading to well below the normal reading, which would, within the pulse oximetry guidelines, have signalled the need to call for medical assistance. By this time the medical consensus had already been reached to take Anja to theatre.

When Anja arrived in the anaesthetic room her respiration rate had climbed dramatically and she had emptied her bowels – another potential sign of stress. Anja was in theatre for some time where it was discovered that she had a 60 per cent stricture of her trachea (**tracheal stricture**). Because of the supplementary oxygen, this had not been reflected in the pulse oximetry recording, which measured the level of oxygen saturation of haemoglobin and not the effectiveness of pulmonary ventilation. Had Maureen relied only on the pulse oximeter readings to assess Anja's well-being, it might have taken longer for Anja to receive the medical intervention she needed. Maureen's experience had taught her to look at her patient as well as the physiological data, and to take note of her intuitive promptings.

The case study illustrates the benefits of nurses integrating their subjective impressions with the available objective data to enhance patient care. Combining subjective knowledge of the person with the analysis of physiological data obtained (e.g. Anja's pulse oximetry readings and respiration rate) is an important part of nursing practice. The subjective element of this integration of knowledge is gained from seeing and examining the person/patient as well as communicating with them and taking note of interactive information. Sometimes the strength of practitioner opinion is enhanced by a consensus decision when other professionals are consulted, in order to ascertain whether they have come to the same conclusions given the same information (for more on this, see Chapter 6).

Making sense of subjective evidence is a part of developing your learning of nursing. Learning a skill means transforming information into embedded knowledge, which is manifested through intuitive and skilled action – what some call *craftsmanship* (Sennett, 2008). Learning the craft of nursing will inevitably be based on your personal experiences, opportunities and motivations, such as curiosity to find out more, which develops into the practical knowledge of nursing – what some call *the professional craft* (Titchen, McGinley and McCormack, 2004, p108). Consider the following case study to understand the role of subjectivity in the development of practice.

CASE STUDY: Sunitta's developing practice

Sunitta was in the first year of her nurse preparation programme and was trying to develop her practice. She had little experience in care settings, but came from a large extended family with whom she interacted a lot. Sunitta's mentor was impressed with her ability to develop a therapeutic relationship with her patients. Sunitta would introduce herself and with an easy manner find out what they needed most. As she became more confident, Sunitta was able to deal with more challenging situations such as working with a confused patient. However, Sunitta found it difficult to deconstruct what she did so fluently in practice in order to identify what it was that she did and ways of improving it.

In order to provide evidence of how she was developing her practice of establishing therapeutic relationships, Sunitta needed to find a way to demonstrate how her practice was changing. Sunitta made use of a reflective approach that allowed her to use stories of her practice, which she then examined through reflective writing (you are referred to the book *Reflective practice in nursing* in this series to find out more about this). Critically examining these stories in relation to communication theory helped Sunitta to develop her understanding of possible alternative strategies that she might use should the situation demand it. She also became clearer about how her communication responses were triggered and what she found difficult, which was a first step to being able to employ alternative strategies.

Discussing her practice experiences with others during an action learning set on her return to university helped Sunitta to identify some further ways of responding that some of her peers had used. One peer had needed to deal with conflict when a patient became very angry. Sunitta found this account especially helpful as she knew that conflict was something she avoided. She decided to return to the literature to find out more and to talk to her mentor about this the next time she was in practice.

This case study helps to illustrate the importance of recognising the contribution of personal as well as professional experiences in the development of subjective knowledge for practice. Private and professional knowledge interrelate and continue to develop and become transformed as they become integrated, informing each other and making something new. Nevertheless, it is also important to validate this knowledge. Sunitta did this by reading communication literature and through discussion with her mentor. This is important in order to be able to articulate new knowledge.

What patients find helpful in the relationships they build with nurses is not always easy to research and therefore the evidence of what works must be subjectively grasped (Baines, 1998). Developing relationships for good practice can relate to how cared for individuals feel themselves to be. It is of note that despite increasing scientific certainty, some recent patient experiences of healthcare are much more negative in terms of standards of care (Patients Association, 2009), suggesting that best evidence needs to also translate into understanding the subjective experience of care. This is because nursing practice is reliant on the subjective understanding of the person undertaking the practice as well as their interpretations of the evidence their practice is based upon.

Implementing best evidence through technological processes can sometimes lead to intimacy becoming lost, reducing opportunities for subjective assessment of patients and developing the *professional craft* knowledge so important to making subjective sense of evidence.

Different types of subjectivities start to emerge from the complexity of people's lives. The cultural subject emerges from expressions of beliefs, values and group norms (Jarvis, 2006). What kind of student nurse you are and how you think is defined in part by your biography, but also through existing as a student nurse in the professional world of nursing. Similarly, patients will be defined by their own histories and cultures, but also through the experience of being a patient in the context of the care setting.

These can all be influential on the care experience. People are *knowledgeable agents* interpreting their existence (Giddens, cited in Delanty and Strydom, 2003, p378). Therefore, any interpretations people apply to their experience will by their very nature be unique and consequently difficult to explain to others. Observed behaviours do not tell the whole story as people adapt what they are doing moment by moment in response to how they interpret their world, which is subjective. The **Hawthorne effect** – where behaviours change because people know they are being observed – is one example of the limitations that may arise with evidence that claims to be objective but ignores the importance of relationships and interaction between people (Barker, 2010). A subjective account is more revealing because of 'insider knowledge' than an account by someone trying to interpret or translate that experience into a more generalisable form (West et al., 2007). What this suggests is that practitioners need to consider how sufficient their insight of patient experience is and what this is based upon. You may want to work through the following scenario to help you to understand the difference between insider knowledge and that of someone trying to understand their experience from the outside.

Activity 5.1	Critical thinking

Brigid was a lady in her 30s who worked in an office. Four years ago she had noticed a loss of sensation in her right leg that made walking cumbersome at times. This persisted for three weeks and then went away. It recurred in her other leg a year later and again lasted for only a few weeks. Brigid noticed that she was also tired during these episodes. Her doctor could find little wrong and assumed Brigid was stressed.

Brigid knew her own body and still had a nagging sense that something was wrong. She did not think that work was particularly stressful at the times the loss of sensation occurred. She noted that the loss of sensation also varied in intensity, becoming worse when she had a bath. Brigid felt that her doctor did not believe her and this made it harder for her to catalogue and report her symptoms accurately.

How might you help to make sense of Brigid's experience?

There is an outline answer to this question at the end of the chapter.

Patients have a better understanding of what an illness or disease process feels like than the healthcare practitioners who look after them – we can only measure the signs of disease but need patients to tell us what the symptoms are. The nature of health knowledge is not exclusive to professionals (Pattison, 2001). It is important that nurses try to employ methods that can tap into this patient understanding in order to identify how their interventions might be experienced by patients.

Objective data can provide information about physiological responses, but how a person experiences their body and changes within it will always be subjective. Through sharing practice issues and reflecting on their practice – as explained in the book *Reflective practice in nursing* in this series – practitioners are able to advance their practice knowledge in subjective ways that interrogate and analyse what knowledge is based upon and how others interpret it.

Reflexivity, based on reflecting on their subjective insights, is how nurses can critically explore the organisations and structures within which they exist and consider what influence they might have to change their situation or be changed by it (Merrill and West, 2009). The critically **reflexive** practitioner utilises four strategies for developing knowledge (Brookfield, 2005). These include engaging with their historical experience, reading and understanding literature, and reflecting on practice and social interaction. Literature can set the experience within a body of knowledge that might include research studies as well as other practitioner accounts that are instrumental in validating experience. Being reflexive involves focusing on opportunities for learning by inter-rogating subjective perceptions, and considering issues of power and how people are thought of or spoken about.

Critical reflexivity means considering what is being asked and how this might translate into personal practice and how this relates to the evidence available in different forms. This reflexive stance offers an opportunity to examine our assumptions and how we might be implicated in the structures that we create in everyday working (Bolton, 2010). Making sense of subjective experience involves understanding how this has evolved over time, how it fits with the experiences of others, what the study of experiences has revealed and what actually happens in practice.

Healthcare is constantly changing, and as nurses we are faced with new knowledge every day. Responding reflexively to changes in knowledge involves being open to experience and re-evaluating what might have been viewed as *fixed bodies of knowledge* (West et al., 2007, p18) – in other words, appraising the evidence of what knowledge already exists and why it might need to change and examining its relevance and potential effectiveness for our practice and how we might use it. This strongly reflects many of the dispositions and influences on practice identified in Figure 1.1 on page 16, which you may like to revisit in order to help contextualise the current discussion.

Such reflexive consideration may lead to new insights into assumptions about how knowledge is used and how practitioners may be instrumental in developing evidence through their reworking of knowledge. Reflexive evaluation is an important method for transforming personal viewpoints in positive ways (Cangelosi, 2008).

If experience is founded on rigorously tested knowledge, then it might be argued that intuition will also be research-based because the resulting knowledge derives from applying research evidence to practice through the mediums of reflection and reflexivity. For example, when thinking about handwashing there is a wealth of research evidence that identifies best practice for completing this, but until subjective sense is made of the actions and steps, the process will not be embedded into regular practice, or possibly even be adhered to. There are factors that may intervene – for example, physical states such as skin allergies and psychological factors such as resistance and stress (Elliott, 2009). In order for practice to become evidence-based, it is necessary to first make subjective sense of evidence by being reflexive. Completing Activity 5.2 might help you to identify how to develop some critical reflexivity.

Activity 5.2   *Critical thinking*

Think about what you know about nutritional care by considering the following questions.

- What do you know about nutritional care?
- How have you developed this knowledge?
- Has this knowledge changed at all and if so how?
- How important is it to you to keep this knowledge updated?
- What might you do about updating your knowledge?
- What might prevent you from updating your knowledge?
- What might be the consequences of updating/not updating your knowledge, to the patient, to you, to the profession, to the organisation?

There is an outline answer to this activity at the end of the chapter.

Relating subjective experience to other forms of evidence

Subjectivity may be constrained into a more acceptable form by dominating factors such as policy and procedures (West et al., 2007). Underpinning the drive for modernisation of the health service is the commitment to improving quality, and evidence-based practice is viewed as one way to help achieve this (Craig and Smyth, 2002). In this way it becomes possible to identify what decisions are based upon and their potential outcomes. Qualitative research aims to find contextual and personal explanations for phenomena while quantitative research aims to measure and record instances and events. Nevertheless, quantifying reality alone can miss cues that help to extend the understanding of events, particularly from the patient's perspective. Such aspects may include attitudes, beliefs, thinking and feeling. Who, why, where and when are the questions of the qualitative thinker (Janesick, 2003) and can be seen to link to those of critical reflexivity as detailed earlier. Asking how people are feeling is also important to help understand effects. Such questioning is essential to ensure that you are always challenging your own practice and relating to the evidence available for what you are doing.

Some forms of research try to categorise and predict what sometimes might be more confused and subjective. For example, it may be possible to predict how a person is likely to react to a particular medication, but how that medication makes someone actually feel is likely to vary from person to person and this may influence their compliance with a treatment regimen, which will ultimately influence its effectiveness. In nursing, we are dealing with unique human beings making subjective experience important for consideration. Illness is a **phenomenological** experience (Carel, 2008). For example, feeling pain is a very subjective experience, and although pain assessment tools may be able to categorise levels, the actual intensity of the experience remains subjective (Buswell, 1998). Undertaking Activity 5.3 might help you to consider ways in which understanding the client perspective might be important and relevant to your practice.

Activity 5.3   *Reflection*

Think about how pain is measured in your present or recent placement. What evidence supports this measurement? Now think about what prompts you to administer pain medication. Now think about a time when you experienced significant pain. Was there any alteration to the way you approached patients in practice following your subjective experience and if so, how?

There is an outline answer to this activity at the end of the chapter.

How we react as individual nurses to different situations is relevant to the learning that we take from those experiences. In some mainstream research traditions people are viewed as cognitive information-processing subjects, missing the more intimate and diverse factors of learning such as the emotional and biographical (West et al., 2007). What this means is that people may focus on functional understanding and consequently miss subjective knowledge that is part of the lived embodied experience from which processes and interactions arise. Nevertheless, there is also a danger in assuming that subjective experience and acting on intuitive knowing is enough. It is likely that you will have come across the expressions 'We have always done things this way' or 'I know from experience'. The danger with this is that it is someone else's experience; your interpretation or level of experience may not be identical to theirs and therefore the results of your actions may not be identical either.

A range of evidence is required in order to choose the most appropriate action for the circumstances. Hamm's cognitive continuum (cited in Thompson and Dowding, 2002, p13) suggests that intuition and scientific knowledge are at different ends of a spectrum of evidence where judgements are formed using different thought processes. Analytical modes use research and experimental evidence from which to draw inferences while peer discussion invites the experience of others to help inform judgements, and the intuitive mode is based on developed expertise. However, in practice a number of these modes may be in use at the same time within a given situation and, therefore, categorising different forms of evidence in a hierarchy may have limitations. For example, empirical research informs choices in wound management but subjective experience also directs action. Consider the following scenario to help you to identify how subjective experience relates to different forms of evidence.

Activity 5.4   *Critical thinking*

Betty is a woman in her 70s who has previously suffered a stroke that has left her partially paralysed. She is admitted to hospital with a chest infection, but is noted to also have a sacral pressure sore.
    What evidence might be used when managing Betty's pressure sore?

There is an outline answer to this question at the end of the chapter.

Working through the scenario you may have identified that the kind of evidence used for practice also relates to different stances that might be adopted.

Particular stances

Evidence-based practice focuses on the need for research awareness in order to provide good-quality patient care. Thinking about the evidence on which to base your practice requires effort to interrogate the appropriateness of that evidence for the situation. Part of such interrogation involves considering the stance of the evidence and whether it also relates to a medical or nursing model of care. For example, a medical model tends to employ a reductionist, rational approach to finding solutions to medical problems by concentrating on signs and symptoms that enable the calculation of risk and benefit and a generalised response to intervention (Greenhalgh, 2006). In this stance health is viewed from a deficit perspective with problems becoming deconstructed in order to identify potential solutions. Taking such a stance encourages objective decision making, which is an important part of being a professional, but it can also become detached from your and the patient's subjective experience, affecting the quality of therapeutic relationships. Reading the following case study may help to illustrate this point.

CASE STUDY: Breast screening diagnosis

Finnola was in her early 50s when she was invited for a **mammogram** as part of the National Breast Screening programme. She attended for her appointment at the mobile unit and was subsequently called back to the main breast screening unit for further tests. While awaiting this appointment Finnola was extremely anxious and had convinced herself that she had cancer. When she attended for her appointment Finnola was told that she needed to undergo an ultrasound scan and a **biopsy** because there was an area of shadowing in her left breast.

Finnola was seen by the breast physician who examined her breasts and showed her the X-rays to highlight the abnormal area. Finnola returned once more for the biopsy result, which indicated that the cells in the shadowed area were **benign**. Finnola was told that she was free to go and would be called again for screening during the next round.

Finnola left the unit greatly relieved with the benign result and conversant with the clinical explanations, but still rather anxious about whether the abnormal area might change in the future. The interval between screenings seemed a long time to wait and although she remained well, she also remained worried.

The case study may have helped you to understand that while the evidence on which diagnosis and treatments are based needs to be rigorous, there also needs to be some interaction and attachment to the person to help them to make sense of the implications for their lives and to be able to work with the information. Barriers to implementing evidence-based practice include problems with understanding the research findings and being able to translate them into practice in a way that is acceptable to the practitioner and patient (Brown, 1995). Inclusion of consideration of subjective experience can promote human elements that are important to feeling cared for and for your learning.

Organisational models

Organisational models use deductive and inductive approaches to promote adoption and implementation of evidence-based practice (Kitson et al., 1996). The deductive process involves audit and drafting clinical guidelines from rigorously tested knowledge. The inductive process entails observing, interpreting and analysing daily occurrences generating new theory. These methods are useful for formulating policies (Couchman and Dawson, 1995). Policies and procedures can help to legitimate nurses' knowledge (Manias and Street, 2000).

Policies are agreed courses of action that have been endorsed by the organisation, such as clinical protocols or guidelines detailing mandatory or recommended approaches to treating specific clinical problems. Standards provide statements of good practice with benchmarks against which practice can be audited. However, overreliance on an organisational stance that describes what should be done in particular circumstances can also result in formulaic judgements and difficulty when faced with situations that require flexibility. As experience is produced from practice every day it would seem that it also plays some part in generating the evidence base. By undertaking Activity 5.5 you will be able to understand how policies are formed.

Activity 5.5   *Research and finding out*

When you are next in your placement, look at the policy folders or intranet and choose a policy to examine. Consider the following.

- What category does the policy fall into in terms of protocol or guideline?
- Is the reason for the policy explained?
- Is the document evidence-based and referenced?
- Does the document reflect best practice by identifying procedures to be followed?
- Is the policy written in a clear and jargon free style?

There is an outline answer to this activity at the end of the chapter.

Action research

Action research is another inductive process through which practice may be moved forward and involves reflection on practice and description of change potential and problems. The outcomes and claims to knowledge of action research as a methodology are still hotly debated (Kemmis and McTaggert, 2003). You can read more about this in the final chapter of the companion book in this series on *Understanding research for nursing students* (Ellis, 2010).

The **gestalt** moment where understanding comes together is an integral part of this type of evidence that enables the practitioner to make such connections for their own learning (McNiff and Whitehead, 2002). The focus within this stance is on the practitioner's learning. A number of philosophies can inform this approach, including the scientific perspective, interpreting patterns and behaviours, and removing barriers and constraints to enable individuals to change. There are fine lines between routine problem solving, reviewing practice and interrogating practice to develop an evidence base. The nature of knowledge is that it grows, at least in part, from a fusing of objective experience with subjective understanding. Gadamer (1989) describes this as a fusing of horizons from the perspective of the investigator who brings their own preconceptions (current knowledge) to a situation to develop new understandings. McNiff and Whitehead (2002) suggest that it is important to 'organically' grow theory within practice. However, this assumes that practice is the measure of the validity of nursing knowledge.

Both nursing practice and nursing theory are important. Practice without theory may lack direction and could be dangerous, while theory without practice becomes pointless because it remains abstract. Undertaking the following activity can help you to identify how practice might produce theory.

| Activity 5.6 | Reflection |

Think about what you have learned from your practice so far. How might you frame this process to look more rigorously at the evidence base of your practice?

There is an outline answer to this activity at the end of the chapter.

Making sense of your practice means also contextualising the lived experience of the practitioner and the patient being cared for.

Contextualising lived experience

It is important to be able to integrate theory with the lived experience of practice in order to be able to focus upon what evidence is needed and how it is used. Making sense of the evidence base from different stances is likely to be achieved through engagement with intellectual activities to support creativity in nursing practice, and development and innovation.

Fasnacht (2003, p196) claims that nursing's interpretation of creativity is expressed in terms of the 'product' rather than the 'processes'. The product referred to here is that of nursing outcomes as opposed to the process of the nursing care. However, it could be suggested that it is necessary to have a goal in order to develop a process that enables you to reach it. Making sense of subjective experience is part of this process. It could be contended that without an understanding of patient experiences and concerns (as they are the end users of healthcare), education and practice remain sterile and unrelated, and the evidence base for practice is harder to grasp. As patient care crosses many professional boundaries, these experiences are better considered holistically, rather than examined as fragments that may omit important professional insight.

Experience is produced from practice and records the outcome of that practice. Contextualising and making sense of subjective experience involves thinking about the human factors inherent in practice and how these might be influential to and influenced by different forms of enquiry. The process is illustrated in Figure 5.1.

Figure 5.1: The process of understanding the context of evidence

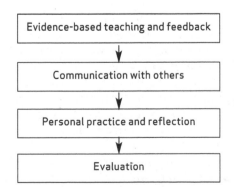

Constantly reflecting on our practice and evaluating processes that are successful and those that are less so will help alert us to how our practice is evolving. Methods that can add rigour to processes of reflection and evaluation are clinical supervision and critical reflection as explained in the book *Reflective practice in nursing* in this series. Such evaluation involves comparing the evidence of successful interaction and intervention with alternatives, to help plan future actions that are likely to be effective.

Clinical supervision involves the guidance of an experienced facilitator to add depth to the reflection undertaken by the practitioner. This might occur within practice or the university, in groups or individually. It is also possible to develop a form of peer supervision that involves peer questioning of subjective experiences, interpretations and the actions, decisions and knowledge used to underpin these. However, the rigour of this is likely to be limited by the level of knowledge of that peer and therefore this form of supervision may be more useful to develop some of the questions that you might want to ask yourself.

Making sense of subjective experience also requires evaluating what you read and are told, and how this fits with practice and research findings. Maintaining a reflective log that you discuss regularly with your tutor is another way in which you can contextualise your lived experience within the framework of evidence-based teaching. Used together, these methods could offer a supported reflexivity that can help to integrate subjective knowledge, practice and theory. Undertaking Activity 5.7 might help you to develop some strategies for contextualising and evaluating your subjective experience.

Activity 5.7   *Reflection*

Use the following questions to interrogate your subjective experience.

- What is informing my knowledge and practice?
- How do I feel about this?
- What works well/less well and why might this be?
- What might need to change and how will I do this?
- What have I learned from this?

As this activity is based on your experiences, there is no outline answer at the end of the chapter.

C H A P T E R   S U M M A R Y

This chapter has considered how subjective experience is relevant and might be used both to create evidence for practice and to create a context for other different forms of evidence that may be used for practice. In particular, the role of subjective experience in supporting learning about practice and accessing the patient/client experience as part of identifying the effectiveness of practice has been explored. Different stances may be employed but ultimately practice deals with unique human beings and therefore human factors need to be included. Utilising a holistic approach that is inclusive of different forms of enquiry, evidence and stances will enrich your knowledge and practice within the ethos of nursing.

Activities: brief outline answers

Activity 5.1: Critical thinking (page 72)

Making sense of Brigid's symptoms requires *listening* to her experience. This means attending not only to the physiological effects but also to how she *feels* within her own body. Doing this helps to access the insider knowledge that external measurement may miss. You could help Brigid by talking to her and documenting her experience. This can record whether there is a pattern to her symptoms – or particular triggers – and so start to establish evidence based on her subjective experience.

Activity 5.2: Critical thinking (page 74)

Nutritional care has changed over time.

- Your knowledge about nutritional care may include understanding how to use a variety of scoring systems to assess a patient's nutritional needs and which intervention strategy and referral options to incorporate into care planning and delivery. This might include knowledge of the biological basis of nutrition and different food groups, and of the role of the dietician. Your knowledge about treatment may, in addition to the knowledge already mentioned, include how to encourage patients to eat, understanding the types of diet available for growth and repair and weight reduction, and the different equipment used for line feeds.
- It is likely that you will have developed this knowledge through integrating theory from classes at university and reading with what you have observed in practice. You may have observed a variety of practice, some of which may not correspond with what you have read/been taught. It is at this point that you would need to identify what is the most appropriate practice through reflecting on the evidence base of what you know.
- Your knowledge is likely to have started from the fixed point of the theory you were taught at university. It is likely to have progressed and expanded as your practice has included a variety of patients and clients, allowing you to make subjective sense of the theory by putting it into practice. Equally, new research findings are likely to become incorporated into teaching and organisational guidance, and therefore inform your thinking as you progress through the programme.
- How important it is to you to keep this knowledge updated will depend on your subjective interpretations of being a nurse
- To keep your knowledge up to date you might read journal articles regularly (see Chapter 2 for strategies for identifying sources of appropriate literature) and discuss practice with peers and practice colleagues. You might even be involved in an action learning set or clinical supervision group who could help you with this.
- What might prevent you from updating your knowledge is likely to include lack of time, tiredness, not knowing how to update your knowledge and maybe even a lack of desire to do so, thinking that others know best.
- The consequences of updating your knowledge could be: for the patient, that they receive up-to-date care; for you, that you increase your knowledge and understanding; for the profession, that you are upholding the reputation of the profession; and for the organisation, that it is seen to be facilitating good care. The consequences of not updating your knowledge might be: for the patient, that their nutritional status becomes compromised through ineffective care; for you, that you fail to keep your understanding up to date; for the profession, that nurses are viewed as ineffective; for the organisation, that standards of care are poor.

Activity 5.3: Reflection (page 75)

It is likely that some kind of pain assessment tool is utilised in the practice area. This will be associated with a range of medication and a formula for administration. These are likely to be based on the findings of research studies. However, you are also likely to take note of patient body language and expressions of pain to help guide your assessment of the need for pain relief. If you have experienced significant pain yourself, your awareness of the difference in feeling and experience is likely to be heightened. This may develop your alertness to the variety of pain intensity and subtle signs, and to what questions to ask to help the patient to access the appropriate medication at the appropriate time.

Activity 5.4: Critical thinking (page 75)

You may have identified research findings relating to pressure sore scoring systems and wound management as an evidence base for choosing treatment strategies. The practice area might have a policy relating to the choice of equipment in terms of mattresses. It is likely that you would also have thought about Betty's experience in terms of comfort and pain control, and the evidence that this provided of the effectiveness of the strategies employed. You might also have considered the role of audit in distinguishing the effectiveness of interventions used in your area of practice. Throughout this you might have been reviewing your own experience in terms of what you were observing as helping and hindering the pressure sore to heal. In this way practice can also inform theory.

Activity 5.5: Research and finding out (page 77)

Policies should be complete, yet simple and easy to read for a potentially diverse audience. Policies fall into two categories: clinical and administrative. You may have identified that the information can be divided into three levels: actual policy, applicable procedures and necessary instructions. In terms of evidence the policy is likely to have:

- identified the problem and described the regulatory background and expected benefits;
- described the chronological series of interrelated steps to comply with the policy;
- distinguished who the policy relates to;
- determined related information such as underpinning references and training required;
- identified which parts of the organisation, or which personnel, if any, are excluded;
- identified where specific questions can be referred to.

Activity 5.6: Reflection (page 78)

Practice development needs to be patient rather than institutionally focused in order to effectively address patient care. Therefore, the process might focus on the following areas:

- defining why change is needed and what is desired;
- appraising the evidence that supports or refutes the proposed change;
- identifying achievable and evidence-based change;
- identifying key components of your development and their fit with current practice;
- determining what support structures, outcomes and resources are required;
- planning how your development will be implemented and evaluated.

Knowledge review

Now that you have completed the chapter, how would you rate your knowledge of the following topics?

	Good	Adequate	Poor
1. How subjective experience relates to other forms of evidence.			
2. The role of subjective experience in the interpretation of evidence.			
3. The different stances that might be adopted.			
4. How to contextualise lived experience within healthcare.			

Where you're not confident in your knowledge of a topic, what will you do next?

Further reading

Carel, H (2008) *Illness*. Stocksfield: Acumen.
This book will help to you to understand how important the subjective view is to understanding and listening to patients as a basis for practice.

Higgs, J, Richardson, B and **Abrandt Dahlgren, M** (eds) (2004) *Developing practice knowledge for health professionals*. Edinburgh: Butterworth Heinemann.
This book will help you to understand how different kinds of knowledge relate and are relevant to the practice of nursing.

Jarvis, P (1999) *The practitioner-researcher: developing theory from practice*. San Francisco CA: Jossey-Bass/A Wiley.
Reading this book will help you to develop an understanding of how evidence can emerge from practice to inform theory.

Chapter 6

Working with others

Peter Ellis

NMC Standards for Pre-registration Nursing Education (2010)

This chapter will address the following competencies:

Domain 1: Professional values

4. All nurses must work in partnership with service users, carers, families, groups, communities and organisations. They must manage risk, and promote health and wellbeing while aiming to empower choices that promote self-care and safety.

6. All nurses must understand the roles and responsibilities of other health and social care professionals, and seek to work with them collaboratively for the benefit of all who need care.

Domain 2: Communication and interpersonal skills

8. All nurses must respect individual rights to confidentiality and keep information secure and confidential in accordance with the law and relevant ethical and regulatory frameworks, taking account of local protocols. They must also actively share personal information with others when the interests of safety and protection override the need for confidentiality.

Essential Skills Clusters

This chapter will address the following ESCs:

Cluster: Care, compassion and communication

1. As partners in the care process, people can trust a newly registered graduate nurse to provide collaborative care based on the highest standards, knowledge and competence.

2. People can trust the newly registered graduate nurse to engage in person centred care empowering people to make choices about how their needs are met when they are unable to meet them for themselves.

6. People can trust the newly registered graduate nurse to engage therapeutically and actively listen to their needs and concerns, responding using skills that are helpful, providing information that is clear, accurate, meaningful and free from jargon.

Chapter aims

After reading this chapter, you will be able to:

- identify why working with others in the planning of evidence-based care is important;
- demonstrate awareness of the different groups of individuals that it is important to work with to achieve evidenced care;
- be able to describe some of the barriers to interprofessional evidence-based care delivery;
- be able to describe why service users' views are important in the delivery of evidence-based nursing practice.

Introduction

So far in this book we have explored some of the skills you need to work as an individual nurse providing evidence-based nursing care. We have identified some challenges that might face the nurse who is attempting to provide evidence-based care and have presented some tools for you to take on board for yourself when developing as an evidential nurse who is ready for the challenges of lifelong learning.

Evidently, nursing care does not take place in a vacuum. The complexities of modern care mean that there is a need for any number of professional and voluntary care givers to provide the care that any individual patient needs. There are also care delivery issues that need to be accounted for, such as the experience of care and the individual needs and wishes of each patient.

This chapter will present an overview of some of the issues that face nurses when working with others, including patients. It will also present an argument that working effectively with others is an important element in the delivery of evidence-based nursing care. As in the rest of the book, the issues here are that no single element of care can be considered on its own and that one element of the caring process does not take precedence over another. Rather, the argument about evidence-based care presented in this book frames evidence-based nursing as the delivery of holistic, multi-faceted and multi-professional care, which is supported by lifelong learning, moral activity, reflection and reflexivity as well as an understanding of research, experiential elements of learning and, above all, the needs and wishes of the individual patient.

It is plain to see that the argument made here is quite complex. It is an argument that responds to some of the greyness existing at the boundaries of theory and practice, and, it is hoped, prepares or further develops the ability of nurses to advance the quality of their practice in a meaningful, well-thought-out and patient-focused manner.

Service users' views

Taking account of the views of services users, the patient's voice, is high on the governmental agenda (DH, 2000). This agenda is clearly reflected in the standards for competence and essential skill clusters required of nurses by the Nursing and Midwifery Council (NMC, 2010) some of which are highlighted at the start of the chapter.

What then is a service user? Service users fall into one of two categories: those who are current users of caring services such as health and social care and those who are potential future users of these same services. This explains why the term 'patient' is not used consistently throughout this chapter. In fact, we are all actual and potential users of health and social care (Connelly and Seden, 2003) but most of the time we are not patients and would not necessarily like to be thought of as such. Most of us have accessed care on a number of occasions in our lives, be that because we are ill or because we are being screened for disease or vaccinated against some communicable disease.

What, then, is important about the view of services users about the delivery of care? Clearly, most service users have a limited amount of knowledge about the hard science of care delivery and may not have a view about the quality of X-ray services, the choice of wound dressing used in the hospital or the biochemistry services' use of particular assays. What they – and we – do have, however, is significant experience of how we like to be treated in the caring environment, and how we experience both illness and care. We all also have our own views about the extent of the care that we may wish to receive and how this affects us as individuals.

Activity 6.1   *Reflection*

Think back to a time when you, or a friend or relative, were the recipient of hospital care. What sorts of things served to make your use of the services more pleasant and what things did you think were not so good?

As this is based on your own experiences and reflection, there is no specimen answer at the end of the chapter.

Clearly, as well as the human elements of taking account of people's views about their own care, there are several moral and ethical imperatives that we, as nurses, must take account of in the delivery of care. Perhaps the most important ethical principle, as it applies to this section of the book, is the imperative to respect the autonomy of individuals.

Autonomy is about the freedom to choose. In part the process of consent supports this freedom of choice and involves the nurse who is delivering care in ensuring that the recipient of care understands what is going to happen to them (information giving and individual competence), is free from coercion (undue pressure) and understands what the alternative forms of care are – if there are any (Beauchamp and Childress, 2007).

Issues of both advocacy and empowerment are important to the evidence-based nurse who is focused on delivering high-quality care that is based on evaluated knowledge and is what the patient actually wants. Some definitions regard advocacy as simply the process of representing the views of someone to someone else; for example, Dubler (1992, p85) defines advocacy within the caring professions as *acting to the limit of professional ability to provide for the client's interests and needs as the patient defines them.* In Dubler's view, then, an advocate puts to one side their own view of a situation and represents only the point of view of the person they are advocating for. This view of advocacy actually represents the true meaning of the word quite well as it stresses the importance of only representing the views of the client and no one else. This simple view of advocacy falls a little short of the realities of nursing care, though, in that it makes assumptions about the capacity (mental competence) and understanding of the facts by the individual client. It also misses the point where the decision is tainted by misapprehension or negative prior experiences.

Within this book, advocacy as it applies to the evidence-based nurse is a term used to define a process of representing the views of a service user when the nurse has ensured that they have discussed the nature of the intervention with the service user and have highlighted the alternatives available and the evidence for each potential course of action. Furthermore, the morally active evidence-based nurse will also ensure that the service user has understood what has been said and that they are able and free to make a rational choice about what they want to happen.

Empowerment and advocacy in this respect are seen as different stages along the same continuum of patient-focused care, with empowerment defined as enabling service users to speak for themselves about what choices they have made about their care (Nolan and Ellis, 2008). As in the definition of advocacy the service user must be in receipt of the information they need to make their decision and they must understand the information. This definition of empowerment, like that of advocacy, recognises that the majority of people are able and willing to engage in decision making about their own care. Both definitions further recognise that this is the patient's right and that some people will choose to exercise it and others will not or, indeed, cannot.

Activity 6.2   *Reflection*

Return to the model of evidence-based nursing presented in Chapter 1 (see Figure 1.1 on page 16) and reflect on the nature of the process of decision making advocated there. Identify especially the ethical elements of the model and the elements that apply to decision making that take into account patient preferences and the dispositions of the evidence-based nurse that are 'other regarding'. How do you see these as contributing to user consultation as highlighted in this section?

There are some possible answers and thoughts at the end of the chapter.

Service users' views also extend to understanding the views of individuals – and groups of individuals – who are not currently in receipt of care. These views help to shape our understanding of the context within which care is received and therefore how it might best be delivered.

On a macro level these views are sought through governmental and local authority consultation while more disease-specific groups might be a source of understanding and knowledge about specific elements of care services delivery. In her report on privacy and dignity in hospitals, the Chief Nursing Officer for Great Britain reported on consultations with over 2,000 patients who viewed the cleanliness of hospitals as their number one priority, with issues such as 'having information' and 'thoughtful staff' also high on their list of priorities (DH, 2007). The Cancer Partnership Project – a joint venture between Macmillan Cancer Relief and the Department of Health that consulted widely among professionals and cancer sufferers on the provision and delivery of cancer services – was regarded as a successful model of consultation and led to effective changes in cancer care provision in the UK (Sitzia, Cotterell and Richardson, 2004).

More locally, patient groups, such as hospital-affiliated kidney or cardiac patients' associations, play a useful role in identifying areas of concern for patients and care providers as well as in supporting changes to care delivery.

What is evident is that a move away from professional-driven care has occurred in the UK and that the voice of patients is increasingly being heard.

Activity 6.3   Communication

Next time you are in practice, spend some time talking to some patients about their experience of the care that they are receiving. Make quite sure that they understand that it is their experience of their care that you are interested in and that there will be no adverse affects on their care as a result of their discussion with you. Reflect on what they are telling you about the care that they are receiving and compare this to the answers that you gave for Activity 6.1.

As this activity is based on your own discussion with patients and your own reflections from Activity 6.1, there are no specimen answers at the end of the chapter.

Evidence operates at two levels. At the first level it provides evidence for care in its own right. That is to say, the experience of the patient, the symptoms they express and their interpretation of the care they receive provide evidence for nursing. For example, only the patient can know if they feel pain, are upset or anxious – as nurses we cannot directly measure these. We cannot validate these symptoms through direct objective mechanisms as we have no machine to measure pain or anxiety as such. We can, however, use some objective measures to validate what they are telling us, such as noting a rise in blood pressure or that the patient is sweating, crying or perhaps trembling. We can also validate what the patient is telling us about what they feel through our own subjective interpretation and understanding of what they are experiencing on a human level – through common understanding of human experience, what might be called inter-subjectivity.

At the second level, subjective evidence might serve to validate observations that we have made for ourselves using more objective measures. For example, if we take a blood sugar reading for a patient with diabetes and find that they are hypoglycaemic (have a low blood sugar level), we might expect them to tell us they feel tired, hungry or confused.

What these examples show is that in our day-to-day practice we see interplay between what we can measure and observe for ourselves and what the patient tells us. The argument here is that whichever way round the information comes to us – patients telling us their symptoms or us observing signs – as nurses we are often alert to and able to handle the interplay between more than one source of evidence for practice at any one time.

Sometimes evidence can be contradictory: the patient tells us they are not in pain but we observe them wincing or gritting their teeth. On such occasions it is communication that helps us to express our concerns to the patient and demonstrate both our disposition to be 'other regarding' and the advancing influence of increasing 'practice knowledge' (see Figure 1.1 on page 16). Evidently, in this scenario there is also a need to exercise the disposition of being 'morally active' in seeking via good communication to act in what will be in the best interests of our patient.

What seems clear is that whatever we think about the motivations behind the advance of the evidence-based practice agenda, as nurses we practise it daily within our working lives. Perhaps awaking our understanding of what evidence-based practice means for nursing on a more macro scale requires that we become more aware of how the principles of evidence-based nursing practice operate at this micro level to inform our day-to-day practice.

In this section we have identified that user consultation is an important element of the government's agenda and that it is identified by the NMC as a required competency for all nurses. We have seen that there is a moral imperative for the evidence-based nurse to take into account service users' views and that advocacy and empowerment are key strategies for making this a reality of the care process. We have also seen how interaction and exploration of subjectivity enable the nurse operating on a day-to-day basis to be evidence-based in their care provision and that understanding how this operates might help us to understand the importance of evidence-based practice for nursing on a much broader scale.

Before we go on to explore further strategies for identifying service users' views, it is important that we identify some of the barriers to consultation that might impact on the evidence-based nurse.

Barriers to patient consultation

By understanding the potential problems we are better able to understand how something might be made to work better. We have identified that user consultation takes place at two key levels: at the one-to-one level, where the concern is the care of an individual; and at the group level, where the concern is the general care provided to a group of patients. We will examine some of the barriers to effective consultation at each of these levels.

Communication and interaction with patients are the cornerstone of good nursing care. Communication is time-consuming, however, and the sharing of information and ensuring that information is understood can take precious time out of the nurse's day. Information and frank and open discussion are not easy to undertake in the ward environment where there are distractions and the very real possibility that a consultation will be overheard by others. Our own lack of knowledge and a fear of demonstrating this to patients may make some nurses feel uncomfortable about discussing options for care.

As well as physical and personal barriers to communication and consultation, there are barriers that are created because of the position we hold, or feel we hold, in the multi-disciplinary team. This may lead some nurses to be coy about discussing possibilities of care with patients because they feel that ultimately someone else will make the decision about care. At other times we may feel unable to put into language that the patient will understand the various options for their care. We may feel that we are best placed to make a decision about the care of patients, especially where individual patients appear less than able to make such decisions for themselves – as might be the case for adults with learning difficulties.

It is situations like these that highlight the very real need for morality and ethics to feature strongly in any framework of evidence-based nursing. It would be easier to operate in a moral vacuum where we make choices for our patients based on what we think are in their medical (or nursing) best interests (Benjamin and Curtis, 1992). However, such an understanding of evidence-based care misses the point that 'best interests' not only include physical elements but also psychosocial, and perhaps even spiritual, aspects of who we are as human beings (Dworkin, 1993). This highlights the need not only for a subjective and inter-subjective interpretation of evidence but also for good communication and a commitment to morally active nursing, advocacy and empowerment.

Patients themselves may present a number of difficulties for the nurse trying to discuss care options. The vulnerability that may arise out of illness, physical or mental disability, age or language can stand in the way of effective two-way communication.

Activity 6.4 *Reflection*

Think about the last time you had to share information with a patient. What were the difficulties that you encountered? Were you sure that the patient understood what was said to them? Alternatively, think about the last time you went to a patient following a ward round or a consultation they had had with another member of the care team. How did you try to check they had understood what was said to them? Were you able to ascertain whether they understood what was said to them and what was likely to happen to them?

As this activity is based on your own reflection, there is no specimen answer at the end of the chapter.

Other barriers to good communication and taking account of the opinions and experiences of patients include our own orientations to other people and the beliefs that we hold about the value of this sort of interaction. Sometimes we make assumptions about what patients do and do not know because they are not care professionals like us or, indeed, because they come from a caring background and therefore we feel they should know about their own care needs. At other times we make the assumption that because they have been seen by another member of the team that they have all of the information they need and that we do not need to engage with them.

On many occasions, we feel too self-conscious to explore the patient's opinions about their care because their condition is too embarrassing to talk about or we feel out of our depth discussing issues such as death or mental illness. Sometimes the patients' wishes, opinions and experiences take us out of our comfort zones.

So how might we function in such scenarios and how might we develop the characteristics and dispositions of the morally active evidence-based nurse?

Working effectively with service users

In order to overcome the difficulties and barriers that stop us communicating well with patients, we have to take the initiative. It is not really possible to be a morally active evidence-based nurse without communicating with patients about their experiences and their engagement with the planning of care. At a one-to-one level there are a number of strategies that we can employ that will make this role easier and allow us to add being 'other regarding' and 'engaged with self' to our list of personal qualities.

If you feel uncomfortable discussing issues with your patients, set yourself the challenge of facing this discomfort and make a point of seeking out opportunities to interact with patients about difficult issues. When you have done so, ask yourself how you feel. Ask your patient how they feel. What may surprise you is that many patients want to speak about their how they feel and that because you are a healthcare professional they do not feel embarrassed or ashamed to do so. If you are relatively inexperienced, be careful to make sure that your mentor knows what you are doing and is happy to step in should the need arise. It might also be worth discussing what you found out with your mentor or perhaps at university with your tutor or other students in an action learning set (while maintaining patient confidentiality).

As this is based on your own interaction, there is no specimen answer at the end of the chapter.

Overcoming barriers to communication as a student or junior nurse requires us to make time to spend constructively with our patients, and to use this time wisely. Clearly, the personal barriers to communication are ours to overcome. Investing time in reflection, either singly or in a group, is a useful strategy in allowing us to identify these barriers and ways in which they might be overcome (Jasper, 2003). Some strategies towards achieving good communication are presented in Table 6.1.

While developing these communication skills it is useful to reflect on how an interaction went – either alone (perhaps using a reflective diary) or with other people. Of course, the important element of this reflection process is learning from what went well and what did not go so well in order to plan your approach to communicating in the future.

It may seem odd that we concentrate on good communication in a book about evidence-based practice, but there are many benefits that accrue from good communication for both evidence-based nursing and the nurse–patient relationship. Some of these benefits are identified in Table 6.2.

Table 6.1: Some strategies for achieving good communication

- Practise – go out of your way to communicate with patients, especially when the subject matter is difficult.
- Try to find somewhere private to talk.
- Identify an appropriate time to engage in talk and ensure that the patient knows how long you might have.
- Get yourself a chair and sit at eye level with the patient; this demonstrates that you have time and brings you down to their physical level.
- Speak clearly, avoiding medical jargon and the use of metaphors.
- If you are giving information, concentrate only on key messages.
- Repeat the key messages.
- Ask the patient to recap to you their understanding of the information.
- Supplement information giving with leaflets, pictures and models; if these are not available, write your own notes for the patient.
- Paraphrase to check what you hear the patient saying: 'Are you saying that . . .?'
- Encourage questions; do not say 'Have you any questions?'; instead try 'What questions have you got?'

Table 6.2: Some of the benefits of good communication

- Better understanding of the condition and treatment options can lead to patients being more able to follow the advice given to them about their care.
- An understanding of what is going on can mean the patient experiences less pain and fewer other symptoms (Hayward, 1979).
- Satisfaction with care can be increased (Maguire and Pitceathly, 2002).
- Patients are more likely to disclose symptoms, which can lead to improved ability to diagnose conditions (Centre for Change and Innovation, 2003).
- Good communication demonstrates that the nurse is patient centred.
- Subjective data can be collected and used to inform the patient's care.

Activity 6.6   *Reflection*

Reflect on the ways that you know that a patient is in pain. How do you know what the pain is like? How do you find out where the pain is? In what way can you know if the pain is constant or comes in waves? What does this reflection tell you about the importance of communication?

There are some thoughts and a specimen answer at the end of the chapter.

From the point of view of the evidence base of nursing, communication is an absolute necessity. It is the patient who knows not only how they feel physically but also how they feel about their experience of care. Without interacting with the patient we cannot know if what we do as nurses is effective, nor can we know if what we do is appreciated and if the experience of care is good.

Working with other professionals

One of the influences on practice that we identified in our model of evidence-based nursing in Chapter 1 was 'views of other professionals'. As we saw in Chapter 5, an understanding and interpretation of the subjective views of others can add greatly to both the amount of knowledge that we have and also its depth. Working with other professionals is often termed collaborative practice or interprofessional working and implies something more than the traditional notion of multi-disciplinary working which may be regarded as less integrated.

At its simplest, collaboration is about working together, which implies a commonality but not a unification of being; it comprises conscious interactions between individuals in order to achieve common goals, by the overlapping of activities rather than merely working alongside colleagues (Meads et al. 2005). Similarly, interprofessional working has been defined as *how two or more people from the different professions or agencies communicate and cooperate to achieve a common goal* (Øvretveit, Mathias and Thompson, 1997). As such, interprofessional working is seen as being much broader in its scope than multidisciplinary teamwork and is not just about how practitioners work together but rather about how they manage and plan tasks for the benefit of patients, groups or services.

Within the context of this book, therefore, interprofessional working and collaboration are more about who the individual is rather than what they do – it is one of the dispositions identified in Chapter 1 as being 'other regarding', which supports the notion of allowing the views of other professionals to influence nursing practice.

So what are the benefits of interprofessional practice and collaboration for the evidence-based nurse? In the scheme that was presented in Chapter 1, evidence-based nursing is seen as the ability to think judiciously about different strands of information that may collectively be drawn together to create evidence. We saw in Chapter 5 that some of the influences on practice include subjective information and the ability to assimilate this into our understanding of the delivery of care through reflection and reflexivity.

Put simply, the point is this: if we are happy to allow our own experience and reflections to guide the care that we give, then it is perhaps egocentric not to afford this same level of respect to the experiences and reflections of others. There are two good reasons for respecting the experiences and reflections of others: first, we ourselves cannot have experience of everything; second, some individuals have trained in specialist and different areas of care than we, as nurses, have, and this may mean that their understandings of and reflection on care may be more sophisticated and better informed than ours.

This notion of being aware of and open to the knowledge that exists within other professions reflects the nature of nursing, which is essentially an eclectic and holistic application of knowledge that we have gained, and honed, from other disciplines.

There is, of course, a caveat to this acceptance of what others tell us: it must make sense. Like all information accepted as knowledge used to inform the individual evidence base, it is important that we subject it to some scrutiny for ourselves. This is the critical thinking that is alluded to in Chapter 1 and that is discussed again in Chapter 8. This idea of checking also reflects one of the messages in Chapter 5 and earlier in this chapter – that we can use subjective knowledge to validate other subjective knowledge (perhaps other people's views on something we also have a view on) or even to validate more objective forms of knowledge such as the findings of research.

Activity 6.7   Communication

Next time you have the opportunity to work with a professional from a different background in the delivery of care, ask them this simple question: 'What are your priorities for the care of this individual and why?' Then take some time to reflect on what this means for you as a nurse and how what they said contributes to what it is that you are trying to achieve for the patient – or not.

There are some thoughts at the end of the chapter.

In essence, then, failing to account for the experience and knowledge of our professional colleagues shuts the door to a very important avenue of learning, which in turn impacts on our ability to develop a holistic evidence base both individually for the patient in front of us now and more generally in the creation of our own bank of professional knowledge.

As well as the concept of learning from professionals from different professional backgrounds, as nurses we need to continue to learn from each other. The same arguments about why this is important and the need to be critical in our adoption of new knowledge apply here as in the examples of adopting evidence from other professionals.

Barriers to working with other professionals

There are a number of issues that act as barriers to interprofessional collaboration and therefore by default to the development of our own holistic evidence base. These barriers – some of which relate to how we see ourselves as individuals and as nurses and some of which arise as a result of the way in which care is organised – need to be understood before they can be overcome.

Activity 6.8   *Critical thinking*

In order to understand how we see others and how they see us, we must first understand how we see and define ourselves. Take a moment to think about how you define yourself as a nurse, a student and as a person. What words do you use to describe who you are and what you do?

There are some thoughts at the end of the chapter.

We said in Figure 1.1 on page 16 that being 'engaged with self' is an important attribute of the evidence-based nurse. But what does this mean?

Being engaged with self is not only about understanding who we are and where we have come from both personally and professionally but also about understanding our motivations, understandings, biases and prejudices. This is not merely about cultural, racial, gender or disability stereotyping; it is about our disposition towards others. Are we willing to engage with others, learn from others, adapt not only our knowledge but perhaps even our values as a result of these interactions? Or are we unable to see the points of view or the understandings that others have and use these to inform not only what we know but perhaps even who we are?

The NMC standards for proficiency require that we *must work in partnership with service users, carers, families, groups, communities and organisations; work with other health and social care professionals collaboratively* (NMC, 2010, p13) and also that we *must use a range of communication skills and technologies to support person-centred care . . . [and] ensure people receive all the information they need in a language and manner that allows them to make informed choices and share decision making.* (NMC, 2010, p15).

The point quite simply is this: we cannot show integrity in our practice and in our communication with others unless we actually believe and adopt this value of interprofessional and collaborative practice for real. Integrity requires that this is not a charade, as integrity means acting and communicating in ways that we actually believe!

This does not mean that we should blindly accept what other people tell us or that we should allow patients to make what are essentially bad decisions about their care. The evidence-based morally active nurse takes account of many issues in generating a plan of care using both objective and subjective information.

As well as potential philosophical differences in our approaches to care, other barriers can stand in the way of good collaborative interprofessional care, as shown in Table 6.3. The existence of barriers to interprofessional working have given rise to a number of tragedies over the years, including the deaths of Victoria Climbié and Baby P (Care Quality Commission, 2009). (The Report of the Inquiry into the death of Victoria Climbié can be found on the Department of Health website – **www.dh.gov.uk** – if you put Victoria Climbié into the search box.) Clearly, there are negative consequences of not working in interprofessional ways that extend beyond not creating and operating within a holistic evidence base.

Table 6.3: Some barriers to interprofessional working

- Professional rivalries.
- Poor understanding of each other's terminology.
- Lack of trust.
- Professional labelling and stereotyping.
- Traditional hierarchies of care.

Based on the work of Barber, McLaughlin and Wood (2009).

Strategies for working with other professionals

How, then, can we get to a point at which we work in a more integrated manner with other professionals? What benefits accrue for evidence-based nursing practice if we do? The first of these questions is hard to answer because alone we are unlikely to change ways of working, although we can certainly be role models of collaborative practice. Perhaps by answering the second question – what benefits accrue and for whom – will enable us to return to the first question and answer it in a meaningful way.

The benefits of collaborative working – certainly within the scheme of Evidence-based practice that we are exploring in this book – arise out of the improved ability to deliver person-centred holistic care. Consider Activity 6.9.

Activity 6.9   *Critical thinking*

Gregg is a 59-year-old man who has been admitted to the renal ward needing immediate dialysis. Gregg has type 2 diabetes, which has caused his chronic kidney disease. The diabetes is also responsible for Gregg having poor vision and a diabetic foot ulcer.

List all the specialist staff to whom it might be appropriate to refer Gregg, and state why.

There is a specimen answer at the end of the chapter.

What is clear from the answer to Activity 6.9 is that Gregg will benefit from the input of many different professional groups from within the hospital and potentially from those outside the hospital on discharge. The benefit that interprofessional working brings to Gregg's scenario, assuming the ward nurse co-ordinates his care, is that Gregg receives appropriate and informed care and advice from the person most able to provide it. His care is the best it can be, and all the professionals involved contribute to this. At the centre of this care is Gregg, who is supported by his named nurse. This nurse co-ordinates not only who sees Gregg but also, more importantly, the delivery of the care that is advised, not for him so much as in collaboration with him. Everyone benefits, there is reduced duplication of effort and Gregg gets the care that he needs.

How can we as nurses achieve this? Certainly in Activity 6.9 none of this would be possible if the nurse involved was not alert to the possibilities that interprofessional working affords. By role modelling good interprofessional practice the nurse is able to receive information from each of the care professionals involved and use this to plan Gregg's care with him. This receptiveness to the input of other professionals is not received blindly: questions are asked, and the ideas and input received are tested against the nurse's existing evidence base.

This chapter has expanded on the nature and purpose of working with others to achieve good-quality, evidential care. We have seen that there are a number of barriers to working with others, some of which are created by us and some of which are the result of human nature. We have further identified some important strategies for overcoming these barriers and some good ethical reasons why we must.

Consultation with services users has been framed as a means of improving not only what we do but also the way that we do it and the ways in which care is experienced. We have explored to some extent the need for interprofessional working to achieve high-quality patient care given that the care needs of individuals are increasingly complex. We have seen that evidence-based practice requires a patient-focused (person-centred) approach to care and must be ethical, responding to and overcoming the potential difficulties this poses.

In this chapter there are clearly a number of very big challenges that the busy nurse must face and overcome if they are to achieve care that is responsive to the requirements of the government, the NMC, the research evidence and, most importantly, the patients who we are here to serve.

Activities: brief outline answers

Activity 6.2: Reflection (page 86)

Being mindful of the opinions, experiences and beliefs of others is a fundamental aspect of moral and ethical behaviour when applied to the process of drawing on evidence to inform nursing practice. Throughout the book we have seen that the evidence base for nursing is not merely about what we do but also about how we go about our work – how it is experienced by others. Within the model of evidence-based nursing there is a need to acknowledge that not everything we do has a basis in scientific or research-based knowledge and that some of the sources of knowledge we use draw upon the experiences and understandings of others. To achieve these lofty goals the nurse therefore needs to be mindful of others while creating for themselves an evidence base in which their practice can be safely and ethically grounded.

Activity 6.6: Reflection (page 91)

We know that a patient is in pain because they tell us. We know what the pain is like because the patient describes it. We know where the pain is because the patient can point it out to us. We know if the pain is constant or comes in waves because we can see the patient's facial expressions and other non-verbal responses to pain but also because the patient tells us. Clinically, this means that we need patients to tell us about their symptoms.

From the point of view of the importance of listening to the patient in terms of evidence-based practice, the point being made is that without communication we cannot know what is wrong with patients and without communication we cannot know whether what we do has a positive or negative influence on their well-being as they see it.

Activity 6.7: Communication (page 92)

Nursing goals are often quite broad and represent an attempt to attend to the holistic care of an individual patient. Within these holistic goals will invariably sit a number of single and discrete goals that are shared by other care professionals. For example, the occupational therapist may aim to restore the ability to self-care while the physiotherapist may regard their chief aim as enabling the patient to mobilise safely. Both of these examples reflect the overall aims of nursing, which often relate to enabling the patient to achieve self-care safely. On a broader view, all three approaches are about contributing to care. If we look at the subjective validity of these three views on care we can see that there is a fair degree of overlap, which helps to validate the three different, but converging viewpoints.

Activity 6.8: Critical thinking (page 93)
Many of us would describe ourselves as caring nurses who work hard to put others first and achieve good outcomes for our patients. As students we may regard ourselves as diligent, enquiring and thoughtful. As people we tend to define ourselves as parents, daughters, sons, friendly, helpful and loving.

Activity 6.9: Critical thinking (page 94)
Gregg might benefit from seeing the following specialist staff.

- The specialist nurses and doctors of the diabetes team would help him get better control of his diabetes.
- The wound care nurse might provide valuable insights into managing Gregg's ulcer.
- The ophthalmologist would prove useful in managing Gregg's deteriorating vision.
- The nephrology consultant would be able to make informed decisions with Gregg about his dialysis and medication relating to his kidney disease.
- The dietician might help Gregg with both his renal and diabetic diet.
- The pharmacist would be useful in helping rationalise Gregg's medication.
- The renal nurses would be able to discuss dialysis options with Gregg and help him adjust to life on dialysis.
- The renal counsellor might be able to support Gregg in adjusting to his deteriorating health status.
- The social worker could help Gregg apply for appropriate welfare benefits.
- The occupational therapist could help Gregg adapt his home to accommodate his deteriorating vision.

Knowledge review

Now that you have completed the chapter, how would you rate your knowledge of the following topics?

	Good	Adequate	Poor
1. Why working with others in the planning of evidence-based care is important.			
2. What different groups of individuals it is important to work with to achieve evidenced care.			

	Good	Adequate	Poor
3. The barriers to interprofessional evidence-based care delivery.			
4. Why services users' views are important in the delivery of evidence-based nursing practice.			

Where you're not confident in your knowledge of a topic, what will you do next?

Further reading

Goodman, B and Clemow, R (2010) *Nursing and collaborative practice*, 2nd ed. Exeter: Learning Matters.
Contains a great deal of material and activities pertinent to working with others.

Koubel, G and **Bungay, H** (eds) *The challenge of person-centred care: an interprofessional perspective*. Basingstoke: Palgrave.
A comprehensive look at the patient as the centre of the care process.

Useful websites

www.caipe.org.uk Website of the Centre for the Advancement of Interprofessional Education.
www.cipel.ac.uk/dissemination.html A long list of useful papers and journals articles in the area of interprofessional working available from The Centre for Interprofessional E-Learning.
www.who.int/hrh/resources/framework_action/en/index.html Link to the framework for action on interprofessional education and collaborative practice from the World Health Organization.

Chapter 7

Clinical decision making in evidence-based nursing

Mooi Standing

NMC Standards for Pre-registration Nursing Education (2010)

This chapter will address the following competencies:

Domain 3: Nursing practice and decision-making

1. All nurses must use up-to-date knowledge and evidence to assess, plan, deliver and evaluate care, communicate findings, influence change and promote health and best practice. They must make person-centred, evidence-based judgments and decisions, in partnership with others involved in the care process, to ensure high quality care. They must be able to recognise when the complexity of clinical decisions requires specialist knowledge and expertise, and consult or refer accordingly.

7. All nurses must be able to recognise and interpret signs of normal and deteriorating mental and physical health and respond promptly to maintain or improve the health and comfort of the service user, acting to keep them and others safe.

10. All nurses must evaluate their care to improve clinical decision-making, quality and outcomes, using a range of methods, amending the plan of care, where necessary, and communicating changes to others.

Domain 4: Leadership, management and team working

4. All nurses must be self-aware and recognise how their own values, principles and assumptions may affect their practice. They must maintain their own personal and professional development, learning from experience, through supervision, feedback, reflection and evaluation.

6. All nurses must work independently as well as in teams. They must be able to take the lead in coordinating, delegating and supervising care safely, managing risk and remaining accountable for the care given.

Chapter aims

After reading this chapter, you will be able to:

- define clinical decision making in evidence-based nursing;
- identify a range of clinical decision-making skills used by nurses;

Chapter aims continued

- describe how the decision-making skills apply to nursing care;
- relate decision-making skills to different types of evidence;
- apply evidence in planned and unplanned nursing decisions;
- understand professional accountability for nursing decisions.

Introduction

This chapter brings together themes from previous chapters about different types of evidence that inform nursing practice to show how they are applied in everyday decisions and actions. Nurses use clinical decision-making skills all the time but they may not always be aware of doing so. From judging how to approach a patient who looks to be in pain to taking urgent action to resuscitate a collapsed patient, effective nursing decisions are life-enhancing and can often be life-saving. Improving nurses' awareness, understanding and expertise in applying clinical decision-making skills is essential in order to provide high-quality, evidence-based nursing. This is reflected in the Nursing and Midwifery Council's standards for pre-registration nursing education (NMC, 2010), and in a Europe-wide 'Tuning' educational research project that defined a nurse as follows:

> *The nurse is a safe, caring and competent decision maker willing to accept personal and professional accountability for his/her actions and continuous learning. The nurse practises within a statutory framework and code of ethics delivering nursing practice (care) that is appropriately based on research, evidence and critical thinking that effectively responds to the needs of individual clients (patients) and diverse populations.*
>
> (González and Wagenaar, 2003)

The emphasis in this definition that is placed on nurses being competent decision makers reflects a shift in expectations of nurses over the last ten years from practically skilled patient-centred carers to **cognitively** and practically skilled patient-centred carers. This involves being answerable and accountable, being able to explain, justify and defend as necessary the reasons, the supporting evidence and the appropriateness of nursing decisions and actions taken in patient care. It is linked to nursing becoming a graduate profession and to lifelong learning for nurses to update knowledge and skills.

This chapter will describe and explore what clinical decision making in evidence-based nursing means, with reference to relevant theory, research and practical examples. In doing so it will relate clinical decision making to the different components of the model presented in Figure 1.1: 'The influences on and dispositions of an evidence-based nurse' (page 16).

Clinical decision-making skills and associated processes

Clinical decision making is commonly associated with diagnosing illness and prescribing treatment, but it is more than that, because unless you switch your brain off when you go to work in a clinical area, everything you do involves making a decision, for example, how you manage your time, interact with patients, relate to other healthcare team members and carry out clinical procedures. To research nurses' decision-making processes, from 2000 to

2004 a group of 20 new nursing students were asked to keep reflective journals about their experience and understanding of acquiring and applying clinical decision-making skills; this included their first year as registered nurses. In a series of four interviews, ten perceptions of clinical decision-making skills in nursing were identified (see Table 7.1).

Table 7.1: Perceptions of clinical decision-making skills from student nurse to staff nurse

Collaborative	Sharing, consulting and agreeing decisions with others, i.e. patients, relatives, nursing colleagues, mentors, managers, supervisors, other health professionals, and other agencies if appropriate, e.g. social worker, home warden, charity worker.
Experience and intuition	Recognising similarities between present and past situations and being guided in what to do by what seems to have been effective before (and avoiding any previous mistakes), e.g. learning how to attend, listen to, communicate and empathise with others in a relaxed but purposeful way that focuses on their needs.
Confidence	Developing self-assurance from previous achievements, knowledge and skills, plus the strength of supporting evidence that enables explanation, justification and defence of decisions and actions.
Systematic	Using a purposeful, methodical, disciplined problem-solving cycle, including identifying and assessing problems, setting goals and making plans, implementing and evaluating (revising as needed) interventions.
Prioritising	Assessing and managing risks: dealing with urgent before non-urgent patient needs; avoiding causing any further harm to patients.
Observation	Making constant use of senses to look, listen or feel if patients need assistance; monitoring vital signs; recording response to treatment; reviewing results of investigations; reporting any concerns promptly.
Standardised	Applying NHS Trust policies/procedures, evidence-based clinical guidelines and assessment tools, and agreed care plans.
Reflective	Undertaking ongoing individual/collective review of experience to identify insights and address knowledge gaps to inform future care.
Ethical sensitivity	Checking patients are informed and consent to care; communicating 'bad news' sensitively; and maintaining duty of care in ethical dilemmas.
Accountability	Ensuring actions are defensible, are in patients' best interests and comply with NMC *Code*, local policy, relevant legislation.

Source: Standing, 2005.

Table 7.1 implies that clinical decision making in nursing is very complex as it involves continually combining and applying many different processes in anticipating and responding to the needs of those in your care through timely, well-informed, justifiable actions throughout a period of duty. In the following case study, a student nurse coming to the end of her second Adult Branch placement reflects on an incident in which she felt she had to take the initiative to support the wife of a patient.

CASE STUDY: The patient's wife

A gentleman was scheduled for an operation to remove cancer from his bowel and create a colostomy (permanent opening in his abdomen) where a special bag would be attached to collect and dispose of faeces for the rest of his life. He was, naturally, anxious about having such major surgery and his wife came in to comfort him before he went to theatre.

When it was time for him to go, I said to his wife, 'You can go down with him if you like. I'll show you where it is.' I took her along and checked that the receiving theatre staff were happy for her to stay until the anaesthetic was given. When she returned to the ward she sat in a chair by the empty space where her husband's bed had been looking very worried. I said, 'Are you OK?' and 'I'll stick with you for a little bit – it is very quiet, there's not a lot to do now.' She burst into tears, and I knew she needed someone to spend time with her, so I said, 'Look, I'll go and make a cup of tea.' I pulled the curtains round and we had a cup of tea together (I don't know whether I should have had one but it felt more natural having a cup of tea together) and a chat. She told me about him and about herself and her family and after a few tears I put my arm around her. She really was grateful afterwards and said 'You know, I really needed someone to talk to.' I look back on that and I am so glad I sat and spoke to that woman and that I knew she needed someone to talk to. It could be my mother, you see, and I would hate to think that nobody sat and comforted her. It was basic human rights, common-sense stuff. A year ago I might not have done that, but I have grown in confidence.

Applying the ten perceptions of clinical decision-making skills to the case study

It is important that nurses can question, examine, explain, justify and defend their decisions and actions when required. The ten perceptions of clinical decision-making skills identified by researching the developmental journey from novice student to first-year staff nurse – and shown in Table 7.1 – offer a useful framework to analyse the nursing student's clinical decision-making skills in the case study.

Observation: The student nurse noticed how anxious the patient looked prior to surgery, how worried the wife looked on returning to the ward, and how she benefited from talking to someone.

Experience and intuition: The student nurse knew it was possible for relatives to accompany patients to theatre when she suggested it and she sensed this was appropriate as the patient was anxious and seemed comforted by the wife's presence. She also understood that the wife had to suppress her own fears about the outcome of surgery and had nobody else to confide in about this.

Collaborative: The student nurse worked in partnership with the patient and his wife to reduce his level of stress prior to surgery. She ensured that the receiving theatre team agreed for the wife to stay until the anaesthetic was given, and she made herself available to support the wife if needed.

Ethical sensitivity: The student nurse extended a duty of care to include the wife as well as the patient in recognising her fears about the seriousness and longer term implications of his condition. She was aware it was not accepted practice to stop for a cup of tea and a chat with a relative on a busy ward, but she judged it was appropriate as it was an effective way to offer the wife support.

Prioritising: The student nurse knew the patient's needs were being addressed in theatre, she had no one else to prepare for surgery, and she recognised the wife might need an opportunity to talk.

Standardised: Pre-operative procedures (consent, bath, fasting, medication to relax, check identity tag, vital signs, remove dentures) would have been followed, ensuring the gentleman was ready for surgery.

Systematic: The student nurse demonstrated skilful use of informative, supportive and cathartic interventions (Heron, 1989): in enabling the wife to choose to accompany her husband to theatre (**informative interventions**); in acknowledging her anxieties, concerns and need to talk (**supportive**); and in giving her permission to express her feelings by asking directly 'Are you OK?' and then reassuring her that she had time to listen (**cathartic**).

Accountability: The supervising staff nurse is technically accountable for care given by the student, but their main priority was pre-post-operative patient care. The student's sense of responsibility for supporting the patient's wife is endorsed by the NMC professional *Code*, which states that you should *protect and promote the health and well being of those in your care, their families and carers* (NMC, 2008, p1).

Reflective: The student nurse applied **reflection-in-action** in taking the initiative to facilitate the wife accompanying the patient to theatre and in responding to her apparent distress when she returned. Looking back, she used **reflection-on-action** in affirming the importance of supporting relatives.

Confidence: The student nurse had grown in confidence in her decision making and interpersonal skills in recognising and addressing the wife's unmet needs, and achieving a successful outcome.

Activity 7.1	*Critical thinking*

One way for you to check whether the ten perceptions of clinical decision making accurately represent essential skills in evidence-based nursing is for you to observe, interpret and record how experienced nurses, role models and clinical mentors make decisions in caring for patients. Make a list of the perceptions (identified above) and write down examples of nurses' decisions and related actions you observe by matching them to the relevant perceptions. Discuss with your mentor what you have seen, whether the ten perceptions are helpful in identifying a range of nurses' decisions, and where you think your own understanding and use of clinical decision-making skills needs further development. Ask advice on how you might do this, taking into account your level of experience, the needs of patients and the availability of appropriate opportunities.

As this activity is based on your observations, there is no outline answer at the end of the chapter.

The case study illustrates a contrast between nursing decisions and actions that are planned and those that are unplanned. Pre-operative nursing care of the patient would have been a well-planned and standardised procedure, whereas noticing and responding to the patient's and his wife's fear and anxiety was a spontaneous or unplanned reaction applying experience and intuition. The relatively high level of contact nurses have with patients and relatives compared to many other professions means they get more opportunities for both planned and unplanned clinical decision making.

Identify a day in your clinical placement to do a 'time and motion' study of everything you do from the moment you arrive to the moment you leave the clinical area. Take a notebook with you to record events and their duration during your shift if possible so you don't have to try to recall everything at the end of the day. Review the day's activities and calculate how much time was spent on planned (e.g. agreed care plan) versus unplanned (e.g. responding to situations that arise) decisions and associated patient care. Match each example to the ten perceptions of clinical decision-making skills as appropriate for both planned and unplanned care. Reflect on whether the ten perceptions apply equally to both planned and unplanned decisions and related nursing care.

There are some possible answers and thoughts at the end of the chapter.

Sometimes nursing interventions need to combine elements of both planned and unplanned decision making. For example, our duty to ensure patient safety means that potential unexpected events such as a fire, an accident in a clinical area or dealing with an aggressive incident must be anticipated, and contingency plans such as a fire drill must be made, ready to put into effect when required. It is important that you discuss with your clinical mentor what is expected of you and your role in such circumstances. Ask to look at policies and procedures for managing such events so you are familiar with them and take part in any drills to practise procedures and necessary skills.

Activity 7.3 *Research and finding out*

Look through the various emergency guidelines and procedures in your clinical placement and see if you can identify examples of the ten perceptions of clinical decision-making skills being applied.

Identify any of the ten perceptions of clinical decision-making skills that you feel should be applied in all situations (including carefully planned care, spontaneous unplanned care and implementing procedures for emergencies) and write down why you think they are important. Check whether your fellow students, clinical colleagues and mentor agree or disagree with your choices.

There are some possible answers and thoughts at the end of the chapter.

Defining clinical decision making in nursing

Decision making involves choosing what action to take from the available alternatives and then carrying it out. In its most basic form it means choosing to do something or choosing not to do it, for example, washing hands before cooking a meal or not (in which case not washing hands is an alternative action, albeit passive) and saying 'yes' or 'no' when someone offers you a cup of tea. Decision making, therefore, employs thinking skills to exercise judgement in assessing the benefits of possible options and choosing a preferred option that is then acted upon. Clinical decision making refers to decisions made by health professionals in the course of their work in promoting health, diagnosing or treating disease, relieving suffering, and caring for patients. Becoming skilled in clinical decision making requires the application of a range of evidence regarding: patient concerns, physical and human resources within healthcare contexts, understanding health and illness, developing expertise in applying therapeutic approaches, a commitment to enhance the well-being of those in your care, and fulfilling the requirements of the relevant professional body.

Clinical decision making in nursing refers to any decisions made by nurses in choosing how to deliver care to patients for whom they are responsible. The Nursing and Midwifery Council is the professional body that specifies education requirements for entry to the register as a qualified nurse and for maintaining registration status. It also regulates the nursing profession through publishing a code of conduct that nurses must comply with or face potential disciplinary action. For example, it states, *As a professional, you are personally accountable for actions and omissions in your practice and must always be able to justify your decisions* (NMC, 2008, p1). Making the wrong clinical decisions is, therefore, not only harmful to patients but it can also damage your career. Learning about, developing and applying effective clinical decision-making skills is vital for the well-being of patients, and nurses' capacity to demonstrate that decisions are justified. The following definition summarises key elements of clinical decision making in nursing.

> *Clinical decision-making is a complex process involving observation, information processing, critical thinking, evaluating evidence, applying relevant knowledge, problem solving skills, reflection and clinical judgement to select the best course of action which optimises a patient's health and minimises any potential harm. The role of the clinical decision-maker in nursing is, therefore, to be professionally accountable for accurately assessing patients' needs using appropriate sources of information, and planning nursing interventions that address problems and which they are competent to perform.*
>
> (Standing, 2005, 2007, 2010)

The above definition emphasises that clinical decisions:

- are patient-centred in anticipating and responding to patient's needs to address their health problems;
- involve identifying, reviewing and applying relevant information from different sources, for example, observations, the patient's story, clinical guidelines, theory and research evidence;
- require the application of cognitive skills such as problem solving, critical thinking, reflection and judgement in selecting the best option;
- are associated with delivering competent, effective nursing care for which nurses are accountable.

In this way clinical decision making reflects the notion of evidence-based nursing, as described and advocated throughout this book, and these skills are central to nurses' professional identity, as stated in the definition of a nurse (González and Wagenaar, 2003) at the beginning of this chapter.

Next time you are in practice, make a point of noting down all the decisions that relate to patient care that *you* have to make during the course of the shift. Later, when you have some time, reflect on these decisions, try to answer the following questions.

1. In what way were your decisions relevant to the needs of the patients cared for?
2. What influences drove you to make the decisions that you did?
3. What types of thinking skills did you apply?
4. How did you evaluate the outcomes of your decisions?

As in Activities 7.1–7.3, try to match decisions to the ten perceptions of clinical decision-making skills.

As this is based on your own reflections, there is no specimen answer at the end of the chapter.

Applying different types of evidence in nursing decisions

Evidence refers to information that is used to support particular beliefs, decisions and actions. It can be sensory: for example, shivering on a cold day and deciding to wear a warmer jumper. It can be emotional: for example, feeling sad or angry about something that happened and deciding to talk to a sympathetic friend to 'get it off your chest'. It can be practical: for example, when your watch slows so you become late for an appointment, and therefore you decide to reset and check the accuracy of the watch more frequently in future. It can be theoretical: for example, listening to a politician's speech about plans to curb greed and corruption in politics and banking, and deciding to vote for that political party at a general election. It can be technological: for example, needing to ensure information on the home computer is not lost if the system 'crashes' and deciding to install a back-up external hard drive. It can also be scientific, for example, understanding that water conducts electricity and deciding to dry your hands and body before switching on the hairdryer to reduce the risk of an electric shock. In the above examples personal decisions, subsequent actions and their potential consequences are prompted by knowledge and understanding derived from a wide range of information sources or types of evidence. The same is true of nursing decisions.

Earlier chapters looked in detail at different types of evidence in nursing. Chapter 1 summarised these in Figure 1.1 on page 16 'The influences on and dispositions of an evidence-based nurse'. In order to see how different information sources might influence nursing decisions Table 7.2 suggests possible matches with the ten perceptions of clinical decision-making skills described earlier.

Applying research evidence to systematic and standardised decision making

Research evidence is often seen as the essential basis of high-quality evidence-based healthcare because it involves rigorous testing of the validity and reliability of methods used and reported findings, which are open to critical scrutiny and testing by others (see Chapters 3 and 4). This scientific (physical and social) approach to generating new knowledge has influenced the development of systematic problem solving and

Table 7.2: Different types of evidence informing clinical decision-making skills in nursing

Evidence influencing practice	Clinical decision-making skills
Research evidence	Systematic, Standardised
Practice knowledge	Observation, Reflective
Experience	Experience and intuition, Confidence
Policy	Prioritising, Standardised
Resources	Prioritising, Accountability
Patient preference	Collaborative, Ethical sensitivity
Views of other professionals	Collaborative, Experience and intuition
Ethics	Ethical sensitivity, Accountability
Law	Accountability, Standardised

associated decision making – for example, the nursing process (ongoing cycle of assessment, planning, implementation and evaluation of care). In many clinical areas the use of the nursing process is standardised, meaning it is adopted as a framework for all nurses to use in delivering and recording care. To guide nurses in targeting systematic care, the nursing process is often used in conjunction with the 'activities of living model' (Roper, Logan and Tierney, 2000) to assess patients' abilities and needs in 12 areas (maintaining a safe environment, communicating, breathing, eating and drinking, eliminating, personal cleansing and dressing, controlling body temperature, mobilising, working and playing, expressing sexuality, sleeping and preparing for dying). In effect, this is a checklist of basic physical, psychological and social functioning needed to maintain health.

Research has reinforced the vital role nurses can play as advocates of patient safety in hospital settings, by ensuring that medical colleagues adopt systematic checklists. For example, nurses in 103 intensive care units (ICUs) were asked to ensure doctors meticulously followed five steps in order to prevent infections to patients when inserting a central line (catheter inserted in a vein close to the heart) to administer drugs, fluids or nutrients, and monitor or stabilise central venous pressure.

1. Wash hands with soap.
2. Clean patient's skin with Chlorhexidine antiseptic.
3. Put sterile drapes over the entire patient.
4. Wear a mask, hat, sterile gown and gloves.
5. Put a sterile dressing over the insertion site.

(Pronovost et al., 2006)

Within three months of implementing the checklist there was a 66 per cent drop in central line infections. Survival increased, hospital time reduced, care was more cost effective, and after 18 months it was estimated that 1,500 lives and $175 million had been saved because of this initiative (Gawande, 2009).

Look at the five steps advocated by Pronovost et al. (2006) and identify which of the 12 'activities of living' functions (Roper et al., 2000) are facilitated by following this checklist.

There are some possible answers and thoughts at the end of the chapter.

Applying practice knowledge to observation and reflective decision making

While research evidence is usually documented, made explicit and widely disseminated, practice knowledge refers to localised, context-specific skills and tacit understanding, for example, the **embedded** customs and practices that distinguish one clinical placement from another. Practice knowledge includes technical skills such as the dexterity to do an aseptic wound dressing, interpersonal skills in being attentive and listening to patients' concerns, and noticing changes in behaviour that signal someone needs attention. For example, a child collapses, has convulsions and loses consciousness, so through reflection-in-action, you decide to turn him onto his side in a recovery position to maintain a clear airway and to avoid inhalation of the tongue or possibly vomit.

A growing body of research evidence means that it is likely there will be some useful information published in whatever area of nursing you are practising in. However, in order to direct a search you need to ask questions, based on observation and practical understanding of patients' needs – for example, 'What new anti-epileptic medication is suitable for children?' Similarly, if research-based procedures are implemented, their effectiveness needs to be evaluated, and this also requires the application of practice knowledge using observation and communication skills in reflecting on patient outcomes. Through reflection-on-action it may be possible to identify valuable practice knowledge, or skills that are usually invisibly embedded in clinical contexts, and then make them explicit.

Try to keep a personal and professional reflective diary that captures some of the events that shape your thinking and clinical decision-making skills. After a period of time, reflect on how these skills are evolving and the nature of the events and thought processes that affect them. Compare what you find with the ten perceptions of clinical decision-making skills described earlier.

As this is based on your own refection, there is no specimen answer at the end of the chapter.

Applying experience to experience and intuition and confidence in decision making

Experience refers to an accumulation of personal, **embodied** understanding that incorporates an individual's unique interpretation of: their role as a nurse; interpersonal relationships with patients, staff and others; theoretical and research input; and influential life events. Connecting these disparate influences defines a nurse's personal and professional identity, which they draw upon in subconsciously recognising patterns in information cues to facilitate their intuitive judgement. In a sense this is what happens between people who have intimate mutual understanding and, without prompting, know what the other person is thinking or feeling. Developing and confidently using this skill as a nurse in quickly assessing a crisis situation, understanding what needs to done and organising an effective, speedy resolution is associated with expert practitioners (Benner, 1984). This is the most difficult type of decision to explain because it may be based on a hunch or feeling that is only justified where there is a positive outcome (as in the case study on page 70). However, this type of decision is prone to error; for example, you might believe a parent who says her child tripped while playing, only to discover later it was a non-accidental injury from physical abuse. It is, therefore, advisable to test out intuitions, for example, by seeking out a second opinion from an experienced colleague.

Activity 7.7   *Communication*

Test out your intuitive abilities with a group of colleagues at college or in the clinical area.

1. Each person privately thinks of a living creature they feel they can strongly identify with
2. Everyone writes (in BLOCK CAPITALS to reduce handwriting recognition) the name of their chosen creature on the same type/size paper and all the names are put into a hat.
3. Someone makes a list of all the creatures identified in the hat for everyone to share.
4. Each person then privately writes down which group member they feel most closely characterises each living creature.
5. Everyone goes through the list of creatures together to see how many guesses were right and how many were wrong.

As this activity is based on your own engagement with the activity, there is no outline answer at the end of the chapter.

Applying policy to prioritising and standardised decision making

In the UK, the Department of Health (DH) is responsible for identifying health targets and priorities for National Health Service (NHS) Trusts to achieve in improving the nation's health. The NHS Plan (DH, 2000) identified that 75 per cent of deaths in those under the age of 75 were caused by cardiovascular disease, cancer, mental illness/suicide and accidents, so it set targets to significantly reduce mortality rates by 2010. National Service Frameworks established criteria to monitor the achievement of targets leading to reduced waiting times to see specialist consultants and early detection and treatment of cancer. All patients attending accident and emergency centres had to be assessed treated and discharged/transferred within four hours. The Plan also called for more health promotion, such as nurses giving patients information and advice on dieting, exercising and self-care such as managing pain.

Applying resources to prioritising and accountability in decision making

A potential problem in setting health targets that encourage more patients to be treated in less time is ensuring that there are sufficient human and physical resources to meet the increased demand, and providing high-quality care. After all, the health targets are intended to enhance public health. Sadly, evidence has emerged that patient safety and the quality of healthcare received has been compromised due to NHS Trusts being preoccupied with the pursuit of prescribed health targets. In 2007 the Healthcare Commission (an NHS 'watchdog') reported that 90 deaths from Clostridium difficile infection occurred in an NHS Trust during the period 2004–2006. It concluded that the Trust had failed to monitor, report, recognise or respond appropriately to the risks posed by the life-threatening bug as it was not on their list of targets. There was inadequate leadership in infection control, not enough nurses for a high (90 per cent) bed occupancy rate, a lack of isolation rooms to contain the outbreak, a lack of uptake on training programmes, and unacceptable standards of hygiene. For example, patients who had acute diarrhoea from the infection were allegedly told to evacuate in the bed as no one could attend to them, and then they were left soiled for long periods.

The Clostridium difficile outbreak came to light because of high mortality rates. The Trust's senior personnel were held accountable for system failings. Clearly, policy, priorities and resource management by NHS Trusts impact upon nursing decisions and the quality of care provided. However, nurses must also bear some of the shame of the misdirected and fragmented healthcare systems that so badly failed patients they were duty bound to protect.

Applying patient preference to collaborative and ethical sensitivity in decision making

In the circumstances described above, patients' preferences were evidently disregarded as there was a failure to provide them with an acceptable standard of care, their complaints were ignored, and the serious implications of unusually high mortality rates were denied. This is in spite of the fact that the Department of Health and NHS Trusts advocate high-quality patient-centred care, greater treatment choice, invite verbal, written or online feedback from patients about their experiences, and have policies in place that are supposed to deal with patients' or relatives' complaints promptly and thoroughly. It is, therefore, important for nurses not simply to listen to patients' preferences or queries regarding their care but to respond appropriately in respecting their views and addressing their concerns.

In some situations patient preference is not catered for because of financial constraints and geographical variations in policy. For example, new drugs prolonging lives of those suffering from cancer are not available in some NHS Trusts because they are considered too expensive, but in others the same drugs are freely available. Sometimes patients do not want the NHS to prolong their lives and refuse treatment, so healthcare professionals are faced with an ethical dilemma.

Scenario

A frail 98-year-old patient who has outlived all her relatives and friends, stopped eating a week ago and says she does not want to be fed by any alternative means offered. If the healthcare team do not intervene, they will be respecting her wishes but contributing to her starvation and potential premature death. If they decide to feed her with supplements via intravenous infusion, they will be going against her wishes but will probably extend her sad and lonely life.

Activity 7.10   *Reflection*

If you were a member of the healthcare team in the case study above, which of the two options would you support and what reasons can you give to justify your choice of action?

The actual answer reached by the team is referred to in the next section for your information.

Sometimes patients take more direct action to end their lives. For example, a young man being treated for depression in an acute mental health unit says goodnight to the new night nurse and goes to bed. When the nurse goes round checking on patients an hour later he discovers the young man dead underneath the covers having tied a plastic bag over his head. The nurse feels terribly guilty for not taking more time to talk to the patient and for not checking on him sooner. These feelings are exacerbated as the police and coroner investigate the death (ruling out homicide), by the parents' grief at losing their son when they thought he was being safely looked after, and in having to describe and explain his actions to hospital managers.

Activity 7.11 *Reflection*

Do you agree with the nurse that he could have prevented the young man's suicide if he had been more vigilant? Do you think the nurse was particularly negligent in the standard of care offered? What evidence might have been helpful in alerting the nurse to observe the young man closely?

There are some possible answers and thoughts at the end of the chapter.

Applying the views, experience and intuition of other professionals (and patients) to collaborative decision making

The dilemma in the scenario concerning an elderly lady refusing food requires careful consideration and collaboration between the patient, nurses, doctors and managers. One nurse had formed a good relationship with the patient through spending time with, listening and talking to her about her past, how she is feeling now, her likes and dislikes, and her refusal to accept nutrients. Sometimes the lady agreed to sip a cup of tea or, with encouragement, to nibble on a biscuit, but it was not enough to sustain her. In contributing to a team discussion the nurse said she did not agree with intravenous feeding because it would upset the lady and deny her the dignity of choosing how to spend the remainder of her life. Others felt uncomfortable that this could be seen as neglect and that every effort should be made to keep her alive. Some wondered whether the lady might not be mentally competent to make a decision and thought the team ought to make one for her in the absence of relatives. However, the nurse argued that the lady was quite lucid, not confused, sad but not severely depressed, and it would be uncaring to force her into actions that would prolong her life against her wishes. The team finally agreed that they would respect the patient's wishes by not feeding her artificially (intravenously) but that the nurses would continue offering her food and drink, and someone to talk to. Pooling experiences and views to debate patient care in this way is a valuable way of promoting effective teamwork, learning from different perspectives and disciplines, feeling valued and recognised by interprofessional colleagues, and co-ordinating and integrating an effective system of care delivery tailored to the individual patient's unique needs.

Activity 7.12 *Research and finding out*

Research the Tony Bland case (the case of a young man in a coma from crush injuries from the Hillsborough Football Stadium disaster in 1989), which set a legal precedent classifying artificial nutrition as medical treatment that doctors (in collaboration with others) could decide whether to give or not. The House of Commons Medical Treatment (Prevention of Euthanasia) Bill (2000) is a useful information source.

As this activity involves your own research, there is no outline answer at the end of the chapter.

Applying ethics to ethical sensitivity and accountability in decision making

As described in Figure 1.1 on page 16, ethical principles (respect for human rights, commitment to good practice, avoidance of harm and treatment of all patients fairly) underpin high-quality, patient-centred, evidence-based nursing. As referred to earlier in this chapter, the NMC is the professional body that sets out the ethical code of conduct that nurses in the UK must comply with. Good practice – for example, the student nurse being sensitive to the wife of a cancer patient in the first case study in this chapter – exemplifies the application of ethical principles, while poor practice – for example, patients being left in badly soiled bed-linen – is in breach of all the above principles, and the NMC *Code* (2008). In order to maintain public trust and the right to remain on the nursing register, nurses must always conduct themselves in a caring, professional, well-informed and competent manner. Where this is found not to be the case nurses are held to account for their behaviour and disciplined, which can include being removed from the NMC register and forfeiting the right to work as a registered nurse.

CASE STUDIES: Examples of misconduct

These are examples of nurses who were removed from the NMC register between November 2009 and February 2010 when impairment of their fitness to practise and/or professional misconduct was judged proven.

- A theatre nurse did not properly check that all instruments were accounted for following an operation, which subsequently resulted in the patient needing to have further surgery to remove a pair of seven-inch forceps left in the abdomen during the previous operation.
- A learning disabilities nurse, employed as a care home manager, acted dishonestly by instructing a healthcare assistant to shred and destroy documentary records of residents' care between March 2007 and April 2008 in contravention of Care Home Regulation Act 2001.
- A mental health nurse threatened to make a patient (diagnosed as suffering from schizophrenia) eat his own faeces and then put faeces in the patient's mouth after discovering that the patient had defecated in the corridor when he found that the toilets were not working.

www.nmc-uk.org/Hearings/Hearings-and-outcomes/

Applying law to accountability and standardised decision making

The NMC is empowered under the terms of Nursing and Midwifery Order 2001 legislation to safeguard the health and well-being of the public and regulate the profession. Similarly, nursing students have to demonstrate good health, good character and fitness to practise, and to declare any police cautions, charges or criminal convictions to ensure patients are protected (NMC, 2009a).

The law, specifically the Health and Safety at Work Act 1974 (Health and Safety Executive, 1974) can protect all nurses in the workplace by requiring employers to take measures (training, equipment, procedures) to control risks to their health and safety. Employees also have a responsibility to report safety concerns; arguably, the nurses at the NHS Trust referred to earlier had sufficient grounds to report serious health risks regarding infection-control systems, procedures and associated staffing problems.

The law can also be used to protect all patients. For example, the Data Protection Act, 1998 (OPSI, 1998) requires confidential patient information to be kept securely and accessed only by authorised personnel. Nurses need to think about the implications of this legislation in their everyday practice, for example, when asking patients about their personal details, given the rise in identity fraud.

Scenario

A patient attends an outpatient clinic for an appointment with a consultant to review recent tests of her heart and lung function. The waiting room is full of other patients, but the experienced nurse loudly and unceremoniously asks her to confirm her full name, address, date of birth, telephone number, work contact details and next of kin, then weighs her and announces the result for all to hear.

It would be more prudent and dignified for the interview described in the scenario above to be conducted privately.

Under the terms of the Freedom of Information Act, 2000, the public have the right to see any records made by nurses or others regarding their care. Hence, it is important for nurses to remember that relevant sections of case notes and reflective portfolios they have compiled could be accessed and scrutinised by patients and their legal representatives.

Some laws relate to specific groups of service users. For example, the Children Act, 1989 (OPSI, 1989) specifies that if you have reason to suspect that a child has been physically, emotionally or sexually abused, you must report it straightaway to social services who are obliged to investigate, and if necessary remove the child to a place of safety. With mentally ill patients there may be a double risk regarding self-harm or sometimes a possibility of harming others. The Mental Health Act, 1983 specifies criteria for the voluntary or compulsory treatment of patients according to the perceived type, level and duration of risk to themselves or others, to protect both patients and the public.

Activity 7.13   *Reflection*

Consider the case study where the nurse in charge ordered the systematic destruction of care home residents' treatment records. Why do you think this was a serious and illegal offence?

There is a specimen outline answer at the end of the chapter.

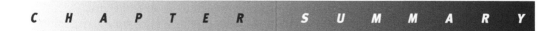
CHAPTER SUMMARY

This chapter has drawn on research into nurses' clinical decision making to illustrate a complex mix of practical (observation/collaborative/reflective), professional (prioritising/ethical sensitivity/ accountability), scientific (systematic/standardised) and personal (experience and intuition/confidence) knowledge and skills applied in nurses' decisions. These were shown to complement wide-ranging sources of evidence/influences on practice using many examples from different fields of nursing.

A high level of patient contact results in ongoing decision-making opportunities for nurses, including planned patient care, unplanned responses to new challenges and contingency plans to apply in emergency situations. Learning to deal effectively with these different demands requires the development and application of different combinations of the above clinical decision-making skills and sources of information to achieve high-quality, evidence-based, ethical, patient-centred care.

Activities: brief outline answers

Activity 7.2: Reflection (page 103)

In reflecting on whether the ten identified perceptions of clinical decision-making skills apply equally to planned versus unplanned decisions, you might have concluded as follows.

- All ten perceptions may apply to both planned and unplanned decisions.
- Standardised decisions more closely relate to planned nursing care, but there is also a standardised option to deal with unplanned situations that you don't feel competent to deal with – that is, to get help from an experienced nurse to maximise safe outcomes for patients.
- Experience and intuition more closely relate to unplanned nursing care, but it is also useful to develop intuitive senses in judging whether planned care really suits individual patients.

Activity 7.3: Research and finding out (page 103)

In reflecting on whether any of the ten perceptions of clinical decision-making skills should be applied in all situations (planned, unplanned, or emergency) you might have identified:

- accountability – as all decisions have to be justifiable and defensible;
- ethical sensitivity – as all decisions should be in patients' best interests;
- observation – to accurately assess patients and evaluate outcomes of care;
- prioritising – to identify and control perceived risks to patients' well-being.

Activity 7.5: Critical thinking (page 107)

In reflecting which of the 12 activities of daily living functions were supported by applying an aseptic technique five-step checklist to insert a central venous line you might have identified:

- maintaining a safe environment – reduce risk of hospital acquired infection;
- communicating – discuss informed consent with patient and/or next of kin;
- eating and drinking – able to administer intravenous nutrients and fluids;
- personal cleansing and dressing – cleaning skin, applying sterile wound dressing;
- breathing – able to administer drugs to regulate heart, circulation and respiration;
- sleeping – able to administer sedatives and painkillers.

Activity 7.11: Reflection (page 111)

In reflecting on whether the night nurse could have been more vigilant, whether he was negligent and the evidence that could have helped alert him of the risk, you might have said the following.

- Yes – he could have been more vigilant as it is never acceptable to lose a patient.
- No – he was not negligent as his actions were reasonable in the circumstances.
- The most important source of evidence for the new night nurse would have been the verbal information received in the handover. For example, he should have been told if the young man required constant observation and then he would have been able to prioritise his care.

Activity 7.13: Reflection (page 113)

In reflecting on the nurse in charge ordering the destruction of care home residents' case notes, you might have concluded that his actions were both serious and illegal for the following reasons.

- It breached the Care Home Regulation Act (2001).
- It breached the Data Protection Act (1998), which requires records to held securely.
- It breached the Freedom of Information Act (2000) by denying accessibility to records.
- It breached the NMC *Code* (2008) and record-keeping guidelines emphasising their value in *supporting effective clinical judgement and decisions* and *providing documentary evidence of services delivered* (NMC, 2009b, p2).

Knowledge review

Now that you have completed the chapter, how would you rate your knowledge of the following topics?

		Good	Adequate	Poor
1.	Defining clinical decision making.			
2.	Identifying different clinical decision-making skills.			
3.	Linking types of evidence to decision-making skills.			
4.	Relating and applying theory to own practice.			

Where you're not confident in your knowledge of a topic, what will you do next?

Further reading

Cullum, N, Ciliska, D, Haynes, B and **Marks, S** (2008) *Evidence-based nursing: an introduction.* Oxford: Blackwell.
Demonstrates critical application of research evidence to clinical decision making in nursing.

Standing, M (2010) Perceptions of clinical decision-making: a matrix model, in Standing, M (ed.) *Clinical judgement and decision-making: nursing and interprofessional healthcare.* Maidenhead: Open University Press.
Integrates professional identity and decision making in nursing.

Standing, M (2011) *Clinical judgement and decision-making for nursing students.* Exeter: Learning Matters. (In press.)
Explores and applies the ten perceptions of nursing clinical decision-making skills in detail.

Useful websites

www.nice.org.uk National Institute for Health and Clinical Excellence website in which you can search for evidence-based guidelines for many different procedures and clinical areas.

www.nmc-uk.org/Hearings/Hearings-and-outcomes/ NMC website link to latest conduct hearing outcomes.

www.patientopinion.org.uk Encourages patients to say what they liked or did not like about care received to inform other patients about healthcare services (also useful for healthcare workers).

Chapter 8

Getting evidence into practice
Peter Ellis

Introduction

So far this book has identified a number of sources and types of knowledge and evidence, as well as ways for looking at and applying the evidence to clinical decision making. Knowledge and evidence are in themselves only conceptual entities; nursing, however, is a practical undertaking and it is important that this knowledge and evidence is translated into practice. This chapter considers how we might become more evidence-based in our individual and team practice.

Getting evidence, of whatever form, into practice is not as easy as using information we know to have been tested to inform our everyday nursing practice. Before new evidence is adopted into practice, there is a clear need for nurses to assess what is already done in practice and how good its outcomes are – we need to establish what we already know. Once new evidence has been identified, the next step is to understand what needs to be done in order to get it into practice.

In conjunction with thinking about the steps that must be taken for a new practice to be adopted, it is important to work out what might constitute barriers to this.

Kitson et al. (1998) identify that evidence is most successfully adopted into practice when the evidence is scientifically robust, it mirrors what professionals think, and it is in line with patient preferences. As well as these issues, Kitson et al. (1998) suggest that the environment of care has to be one that is accepting of change and where there is strong leadership as well as established and reasonable monitoring systems in place.

This chapter will therefore explore some of the psychosocial and practical barriers to the adoption of new evidence. It will explore what might need to be done by individuals and teams to facilitate the successful adoption of new evidence. The potential benefits of adopting evidence in practice from the point of view of the individual practitioner, the team and, importantly, the patient will also be examined.

A model of the dispositions and influences on the evidence-based nurse was advanced in Chapter 1 (Figure 1.1, page 16). This model suggests that any nurse who wishes to act in an evidence-based manner needs to engage with certain behaviours and ways of inquiring, all of which are complementary and supplementary to each other.

Activity 8.1   *Reflection*

Revisit Activity 1.9 on page 17, which asked you to explore your understanding of your own existing dispositions as well as the reasons why you are in nursing. Now that you have read more of the book and have thought about the messages it contains, do you think that any of your identified dispositions or influences are helpful, or unhelpful, to adopting an evidence-based approach to practice?

Clearly, the adoption of evidence for practice has been at the heart of this book. Throughout the chapter you should try to bear in mind that we have so far identified many sources of potential evidence for practice and that the adoption of this evidence will draw on all of these sources to differing degrees at different times.

Questions to ask before adopting new evidence

We have already established that not all information constitutes evidence because it needs to be assessed for its quality before it can be considered as knowledge fit for practice. As well as assessing the sources and quality of the evidence, it is also necessary to consider how well it aligns with clinical need, resources and skills available, how the workplace is organised and managed, and, most importantly, the needs of the clients to whom, and with whom, the evidence will be applied.

These important issues help to ground the adoption of evidence in the realities of practical nursing. Evidence-based practice for nursing is about dealing judiciously with the sources and complexities of knowledge with one foot firmly in the theoretical camp and the other firmly rooted in practice.

Some theorists claim that nursing is an art and others that it is a science. Certainly, there are elements of both philosophies within nursing practice. If the science of nursing is about understanding the biological and physical aspects of care, perhaps the art of nursing is the ability to draw upon multiple and varied strands of knowledge in pursuit of the best holistic outcomes for our patients.

One of the first challenges for nurses attempting to adopt new evidence is identifying and overcoming the real (and understandable if not always acceptable) barriers to change.

Barriers to getting evidence into practice

There are a number of barriers to the adoption of evidence, involving a mix of rational and less rational fears and anxieties. Many of us like to return to places and practices with which we are familiar, things and ideas that reside within our comfort zones. Others are always 'up for' change and challenge, regarding the new and unknown as something to be embraced.

Concept summary: personality types

In one of the most frequently referred to models of the adoption of innovation, Rogers (1962) asserts that there are five different personality types.

Innovators	The first 2.5 per cent of adopters are educated, adventurous and risk takers.
Early adopters	The next 13.5 per cent are social leaders, popular and educated.
Early majority	The next 34 per cent are deliberate and motivated by evolutionary changes.
Late majority	The next 34 per cent are sceptical and more traditional.
Laggards	The last 16 per cent are technology sceptics who do not to believe that technology can enhance productivity.

When managing our own personal and professional development as well as change in others we recognise that not everyone shares the same orientations to change. Nurses, like other people, will adopt a stance to change that is based to some extent on the sort of person they are, their previous experiences of change and their belief in the usefulness of the proposed change and the person proposing the change. Barriers to change therefore arise at a personal, experiential and interpersonal level, and we need to consider these barriers to transition and change before attempting to adopt evidence.

Activity 8.3   *Reflection*

Reflect on the reasons why people do not like to change the ways in which they work and their nursing practice.

There are some possible answers and thoughts at the end of the chapter.

Some of the reasons people do not like to change what they do are deeply seated in our natural desire to be thought well of. For example, if a nurse who has been practising clinically for 20 years is confronted with the need to change a practice that she has engaged with throughout her entire clinical career, a number of questions may arise.

- What is the point of the change when what I do already is good enough?
- If I adopt this change now, am I saying that what I have done to date has not been good enough?
- How do I know that this change will work?
- Do I have the skills to operate in a new way?

These are reasonable questions, all of which may threaten the status and confidence of the nurse confronted by change. These are sensitive issues that threaten to undermine not only one individual but potentially the stability of the team and thereby impact on patient care.

Resistance to change often arises out of a lack of understanding of the need for change. In these instances individuals cannot see that current practice is potentially not as good as it might be. They may also not appreciate that the effects of the change may outweigh the time and energy required to make the change and that in the long run the change may benefit both them and their patients. The need to fulfil their current obligations takes precedence over making changes because the 'here and now' is urgent and change takes time and energy (Nilsson Kajermo et al. 1998; Hilton et al. 2009) and many nurses feel that they lack the skills to implement change (Rodgers, 1994).

A lack of vision and understanding of the change can stand in the way of an individual nurse accepting change. Sometimes this lack of understanding arises out of the inability of a change agent (perhaps a manager or fellow nurse) to adequately explain what they are doing and what the likely outcome is. There is an issue of communication here that will need to be addressed if change is to be managed at team level.

Often there are issues with the way in which change is rolled out. Some team members may feel the process of change has been poorly handled – it is too rapid, or too slow, or communication could have been better. Others may feel that the change is not something they agree with or they may consider that the evidence underpinning the change is incomplete or needs further scrutiny.

Activity 8.4   Critical thinking

What is your personal attitude to change? Reflect on the last change or develop-ment that you had to adapt to. Reflect on your thoughts and feelings about the process, what worked for you and what did not and why. Has this coloured your view of change in the future and of developing as an evidence-based nurse? Why (or why not)?

As this is based on your own reflection, there is no specimen answer at the end of the chapter.

On other occasions the introduction of new evidence is hard to instigate because team members have experienced poorly managed change and are sceptical about any subsequent changes.

The National Institute for Health and Clinical Excellence (NICE) identifies six barriers to change and the adoption of evidence into clinical practice – see Table 8.1.

As well as the barriers to change, there are a number of barriers to the adoption of evidence-based practice that may need addressing. These include the inability to search online databases, a lack of understanding about research, the inability to access research and a preference for seeking guidance from colleagues (Thompson et al., 2001).

If we are concerned about improving lives and providing high-quality care, we need to focus on the shared value of care. Even if our personal orientation is to be sceptical

Table 8.1: Barriers to change (see NICE, 2007).

- Lack of awareness and knowledge of the evidence and changes needed to adopt evidence.
- Lack of motivation both internally and from external incentives.
- Lack of acceptance or belief that the change will benefit patients, that the evidence is good or that it is possible to adopt.
- Lack of skills, or perception of lack of skills, needed to undertake the change.
- Practical difficulties with resources and staff time and continuity.
- Factors in the external environment including the lack of resource and incentives to change.

about the sources of some of the evidence we have to employ as nurses, we should assess the value of the information on its own merit and on the merit of the values that underpin it.

Consequences of not adopting evidence-based practice for nursing

Poor decisions in nursing can affect the quality of life and, indeed, the very lives of the patients we care for. We have identified various sources of information and a number of ways of checking the quality of the information before we accept it as evidence. It is now worth asking the question 'What are the consequences of not adopting an evidential approach to our nursing practice?'

Activity 8.5   *Critical thinking*

Before you go on to read the next section of this chapter, take a few moments to jot down what you think might be some of the consequences of not adopting an evidence-based approach to nursing practice.

There are some possible answers and thoughts at the end of the chapter.

Internationally, nursing is still struggling with both creating and consolidating its professional identity. One of the characteristics of a profession is that it has its own body of knowledge that establishes its credentials and credibility within society. Adopting the broad approach to evidence advocated in this book goes at least some way toward establishing this credible knowledge base, creating and enhancing the identity of nursing as a profession in its own right.

If nurses fail to adopt evidential care practices, there will doubtless be consequences for the image of nursing as a whole. It may not immediately be obvious to some why maintaining a positive image for nursing is important. However, when we think about the need for the people we care for to have trust in what we do at times in their lives when they are perhaps at their most vulnerable, the answers present themselves. Care is best provided and best received when there is trust. Maintaining a positive public perception of nursing engenders trust, and this positive image itself derives from nurses being able to demonstrate that their practice is worthwhile.

Regardless of our professional standing, it remains the duty of nurses to communicate effectively, in a manner that can be understood, with our clients and colleagues. The important message here is that when applying evidence we should not neglect our core activities of care and communication. Rather, the application of an evidence base to practice should be used to supplement and complement what we do.

Adopting an evidential approach to nursing also allows nurses to demonstrate that they are acting in the best interests of their clients as required by the Nursing and Midwifery Council in the code of conduct for nurses (NMC, 2008), which states: *You must deliver care based on the best available evidence or best practice.* Failure to act in an evidential manner in our practice therefore puts nurses at odds with the regulations of our registering body and creates questions about fitness to practise. The competencies and essential skills clusters identified at the start of this chapter require nurses to be competent in care delivery and in the improvement of standards for nursing practice.

Theory

Adopting and adapting to the challenges of evidence-based nursing practice is about the constant improvement of care. Within the context of evidence-based nursing presented in this book, the knowledge underpinning these changes is regarded as having been judiciously identified, conscientiously analysed and proactively adopted. Reflecting on the content of these statements, it is clear to see why evidence-based nursing care is a realistic and feasible route to fulfilling the requirements of both the NMC code of conduct (2008) and the NMC standards and essential skills clusters for pre-registration nurse education (2010).

Acting in the best interests of our clients is a desirable attribute of nursing, although it may not always be clear what constitutes best interests (Ellis, 1996). Whatever view you choose to take of what 'best interests of patients' means, be this improving their health or maintaining their dignity, what is clear is that no patient's best interests can be served in a meaningful way without some understanding of the evidence base that underpins their care. This is not an empty statement since the evidence base of nursing care is concerned not only with what practices serve to make people physically or psychologically better but also with an understanding of how people experience care.

Accountability

The accountability that trained nurses have for the safety and quality of the care they provide can be demonstrated by the adoption of evidence-based nursing practice. Failure to adopt evidence will mean that nurses cannot justify the care they give. While it is true that the obligations of student nurses do not operate at the level of accountability to the regulatory body, they are responsible for their own actions and omissions in the provision of care, becoming accountable for these on qualifying. It would seem sensible, therefore, to adopt a critical and evidence-based approach to practice sooner rather than later.

Accountability is not merely about how we conduct ourselves in practice; it is also about the things we do. Accountability on this level is being able to justify what we do using our professional knowledge, which is drawn down from our understanding of evidence.

As well as our obligations to our profession and its regulatory body, nurses have obligations and duties to their employers. These duties extend to fulfilling our roles as nurses within the clinical governance frameworks established and monitored by our employer and nationally. Clinical governance requirements mean that, as nurses, we need to be able to demonstrate the worth of what we do in working towards the goals of the organisation and in achieving timely, effective outcomes for patients (Scott, 1998).

It seems self-evident that the achievement of safe, timely and effective outcomes for patients is best accomplished by nursing staff who can identify, understand and apply evidence to practice.

Moral imperative

Ethically, it is hard to justify the provision of care that is not evidence-based, where evidence exists. There are many occasions when there is little or no apparent *hard* evidence to support what we do as nurses. This does not, however, mean that what is done to, and with, the patient is unethical. It does mean that as well as striving to do the best for the patient, the nurse operating as a evidential practitioner takes the time to reflect in and on action and adds the experiential learning to their own constantly evolving evidence base.

There is a moral duty on the part of the nurse to use more objective and rigorous forms of evidence to support their practice, where such evidence exists (Milton, 2007). This obligation arises out of the special contractual obligations nurses accept on entering the nursing profession. This contract states that we will provide care to the best of our ability and that patients can expect us to do so, not because we are fellow human beings necessarily (although this is also an important factor in establishing our obligations) but because we have taken on and accepted this additional duty of our own free will.

On some occasions nurses may be required to justify the care they have given in a court of law. To this end it is important that nurses can demonstrate, beyond reasonable doubt, that they have provided the care they can both realistically and professionally be expected to provide. Unfortunately, litigation against healthcare professionals, including nurses, is increasing and it is therefore both necessary and wise to ensure our nursing practice is able to stand up to this level of scrutiny.

The main reason that evidence is important is that it improves the quality of the care that nurses undertake (Berwick, 2003). Nurses should, and indeed most do, take pride in what they do, and this pride should stem from an understanding that what they do is the very best that they can achieve. Providing good-quality care is both good in its own right as well as being important because of its consequences. The key consequence of high-quality care that is firmly grounded in critical and evidential nursing practice is that it improves not only the outcomes of care but also the patient's experience of care.

Activity 8.6   *Reflection*

Try to remember a time when you were in receipt of nursing or any other form of healthcare. How did you feel about the care given and was this affected by your perception of the person/people giving the care? Why?

There are some specimen answers at the end of the chapter.

Managing change and transition

Change can be considered to be an alteration to the way in which something is done or the replacement of one thing by another. For example, a hospital or department may choose to change the type of dressing they use post-operatively, or a ward may be remodelled in order to be able to achieve the Department of Health's single-sex ward requirement.

Transition is an alteration in the mindset of the people who have to undertake change. Regardless of the purpose, or nature, of a change, all change engenders an emotional and psychological response from those concerned. Before we go on to examine the management of change, both in ourselves and in others, it is worth stopping for a moment to consider the psychological impact of change.

Tools such as the Holmes and Rahe (1967) Social Readjustment Rating Scale identify that any life change is associated with stress. Hopson and Adams (1976) proposed a model that explains the changes in self-esteem that people go through in periods of transition and captures some of the reasons why people might become stressed – see Figure 8.1.

This model of changes in self-esteem during transition demonstrates that there is a level of loss and adjustment that is associated with all changes. What the model does

Figure 8.1: A model of changes in self-esteem during transitions, as described by Hopson and Adams (1976)

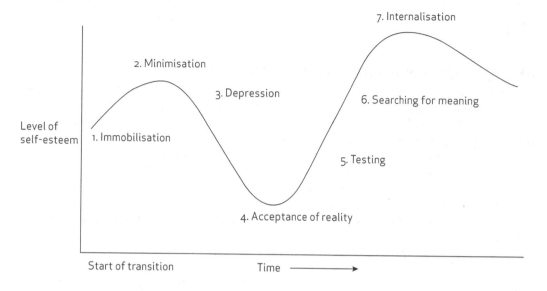

not show is that the transition through the model is not always the same for all people, or even for any single individual. In fact, Hopson and Adams (1976) claim that different people go through the stages in different orders at different times, and that not everyone goes through every stage for each transition they go through. The stages of transition in the model are defined in Table 8.2.

Table 8.2: What the stages of the model of changes in self-esteem during transitions mean

Immobilisation	A sense of being overwhelmed and unable to act when faced with a transition. Transitions that are unfamiliar and ones that are associated with negative expectations tend to intensify this stage.
Minimisation	A coping mechanism when faced with change. Frequently people deny the change is happening. This is a common reaction to a crisis which is too difficult to face.
Depression	People may become depressed when faced with the implications of change.
Acceptance of reality	Occurs at the point when people begin to let go of their old state of being and start to accept the reality of the change.
Testing	Begins when the reality of the change has been accepted. In this stage people start to try out new behaviours to cope with the new situation.
Searching for meaning	A reflective stage during which people try to work out how and why things are different.
Internalisation	The final stage of the process during which understandings of the new situation become accepted. The new understanding then becomes part of the person's behaviour.

Based on the work of Hopson and Adams, 1976.

What these models of the psychological impacts of change and transition tell us is that negative psychological responses are normal. It is important, therefore, that we accept that when we are exposed to change there will be a psychological response, and this is something we should learn to cope with for ourselves, and recognise and manage in others.

Managing change and transition as an individual

As identified in the model of evidence-based practice on page 16, a nurse who chooses to practise as an evidence-based practitioner must first engage with themselves. This engagement with self is about understanding our own behaviours and orientations. It is about understanding who we are and why we act as we do. One of the mechanisms for doing this that has been identified in this book is the use of reflection and clinical supervision. It is only by examining what we think and feel about situations we have been in, and experiences we have had, that we can critically reflect upon who we are and what motivates us. Other strategies have included being more aware of the nursing literature, especially research, and engaging in a meaningful way with it.

Becoming evidence-based requires the nurse to make two transitions. The first of these involves accepting that nursing is about being responsive to new sources of knowledge, new evidence and new understandings. We have to accept that this transition is about lifelong learning and continuing personal and professional development, and that change is an inevitable consequence of working in health and social care.

The second transition involves learning to work with the various sources of knowledge and evidence identified within this book, and understanding how these separate types of evidence can be worked into a larger scheme of understanding. Internalisation of these realities is fundamental to both becoming, and continuing as, an evidence-based nurse.

Activity 8.7	Critical thinking

What are the influences on nursing practice that mean it is necessary to adopt a continuous learning approach to practice? Think about what changes are under way in society at the moment that may result in nurses needing to adapt their practice.

There are some possible answers at the end of the chapter.

So what does this mean for you as an individual student or qualified nurse? There is a real challenge here in that understanding yourself as a nurse will have a direct impact on how you see yourself as a person. Undoubtedly, reflection – trying to make sense of situations and planning how you will act in the future (Jasper, 2003) – and reflexivity – awareness of yourself and your impact on the working environment (Flanagan, 1981) – are skills that are absolutely necessary to function effectively as a nurse in today's care environments. Employing reflection and reflexivity are essential for consolidating the skills and knowledge that you currently have as well as identifying what skills and knowledge you need to develop.

Activity 8.8   *Reflection*

Even if you are the sort of nurse who employs evidence-based practice methods in your work, this book presents a number of challenges that require development and assimilation if they are to enhance lifelong learning. Reflect on these challenges, especially what they mean for you, and devise an action plan for how you might progress as an evidence-based practitioner.

There are some possible strategies at the end of the chapter.

What is clear from this message is that doing nothing is not really an option for nurses who wish to be both patient-centred and evidence-based. The messages contained in this book point to the need to integrate into our understanding of care not only our own reflections but also the views of our patients and insights from our colleagues.

Critical and creative thinking

Critical and creative thinking, as well as reflection and reflexivity, can be used to enhance both self-development and practice. The skills necessary for criticality and creativity are different, but also complementary, and both enhance the ability of the nurse to become an evidence-based practitioner.

We identified in our model of evidence-based practice in Chapter 1 that creative and critical thinking are dispositions of the evidence-based nurse. Throughout the book we have seen examples of creative and critical thinking under different guises in the identification of sources of evidence, in the processing of evidence and, finally, in the adoption of evidence. But what are creative and critical thinking and how might they help us become more evidence-based practitioners?

Critical thinking

Being a critical thinker requires that we adopt the disposition of being inquisitive and receptive to new forms and sources of knowledge. It also requires that this inquisitiveness is guided by explicit reflection and reasoned thought processes (L'Eplattenier, 2001). This means enquiry that is both conscious (we choose to do it) and conscientious (we follow a well-defined pattern of thought). Hence, critical thinking is about clarity and rationality of thought.

As critical thinking is about clarity and rationality, it can help lead the nurse from being overwhelmed with information to a position where they are able to logically analyse and unite ideas from a number of sources into ideas (or evidence) that is fit for both implementation and further analysis. The need for further analysis arises out of the questioning disposition that we identified in the evidence-based nursing model in Chapter 1 and the realisation that healthcare is constantly evolving and therefore our evidence base and understanding of care need to evolve with it.

Activity 8.9   *Critical thinking*

Consider how your understanding of nursing has evolved since you joined the profession. Think about what things you found hard to understand – for example, why there is a theory–practice gap – and then consider what you know about these issues now and why it makes more sense.

There are some thoughts and possible answers at the end of the chapter.

Certainly, the notion of the need for constant and repeated analysis through reflexivity and reflection echoes one of the core messages of this book: that knowledge is only knowledge until something new comes along. This underlines the need for engagement in lifelong learning and continuous personal and professional development.

Evidently, critical thinking is not about the accumulation of knowledge, nor is criticality about being argumentative. It is about strategies that enable us to strengthen and deepen our understandings and develop ideas and theories with which we can underpin practice.

So how can we develop as critical thinkers? First of all, we need to take time to look for and understand the logical connections between ideas. For example, we are frequently told that information giving helps reduce stress in our patients, but have we ever thought about why? Many of us know that stress can arise out of a feeling of loss of control. A feeling of loss of control can arise from not knowing what is happening. So spending time explaining things to patients means they know what is going on, they can make some choices; they feel more in control and therefore less stressed. Next time a patient is angry or irritated by the care they receive, do not jump to the conclusion that they are being rude – ask yourself why. This is critical thinking.

In much the same way, we can solve all manner of problems by thinking clearly and logically, looking for connections between ideas and theories of knowledge that enable us to make sense of what is happening.

Critical thinking is therefore about honing our understanding of an issue by systematically bringing together threads of an argument in a logical way in order to solve problems or create new understandings. A useful metaphor is that critical thinking acts like a funnel, collecting lots of diverse information and knowledge and narrowing it down to something more manageable (evidence).

Creative thinking

For the evidence-based practitioner, creativity follows on logically from criticality. Once we have thought about and understood something, we can decide how we might deal with it. Creative thinking is about exploring possibilities, creating solutions and generating new ideas (Santrock, 2004). Evidently, if we have engaged in critical thinking and thereby understood a situation or scenario, then as an evidence-based nurse grounded in action we need to generate ideas about how we are going to act. Creative thinking therefore feeds into the idea of change and transition.

If we pick up the funnel metaphor once more, while critical thinking narrows a lot of diverse information and knowledge together into evidence, creative thinking may be thought of as more like an inverted funnel, taking the evidence and placing it in among issues such as existing policy, professional and patient preference, ethical considerations and practical knowledge. This broadening out in thinking allows realistic and practical considerations to be made about the application of the evidence to practice.

Creativity is, therefore, the ability to generate new ways of thinking and/or working. This ability arises out of conscientious exploration of sources of evidence and critical appraisal of their worth. Creativity is also an attitude – a 'can do' attitude that says 'There is an issue here where my knowledge and the realities of this situation do not marry up, I will therefore find a way to make sense of this situation'. Being creative is a process in which we constantly seek to refine and enhance what we do, taking into account a broader perspective on practice.

Having engaged in critical thinking activities that identify problems and sources of evidence, we can then use creativity either to solve problems or to improve on what we do. The key to creative thinking is the understanding that there might be more than one solution to an issue that is correct, and that the solutions to a problem might vary according to the situation and the people involved.

This idea of the contextual reality of creativity marries well with the central theme of this book. The reality of providing evidential person-centred care requires us to engage with other nurses, other care professionals, other agencies and, most importantly, with the patient. Engaging with others allows us to see a clinical scenario from more than one viewpoint; it demonstrates the multiplicity of reality and the fact that each episode of care, while often following similar trajectories, is unique.

Activity 8.10   *Reflection*

Some theories of creative thinking suggest we adopt different mental approaches to problem solving in order to gain multiple perspectives on what the problem looks like and what the solutions might be. Using this idea, reflect on a recent care episode from your own point of view, then from the points of view of another care professional, the patient and the patient's relatives. Consider how understanding these different interpretations of the same events might lead you to think creatively about the way you approach care provision in the future.

As this is a personal reflection, there is no specimen answer at the end of the chapter.

Being open to critical and creative thinking, therefore, develops the ability within us to adapt our way of thinking and adopt new practices in care. It allows us to deal with change and transition in a proactive and managed way and generates for the individual the ability to be truly evidence-based.

Managing change and transition in teams

So far in this chapter we have laid out some challenges and solutions to becoming an evidence-based practitioner. In this section we will take the ideas one step further and explore how we might manage the process of change and transition in the team setting.

Getting evidence into practice in a team is all about the management of change, and sustaining the impetus of change management is all about creating environments of care that are not only responsive to evidence but are also environments in which nurses actively seek out opportunities to incorporate evidence into their day-to-day practice.

Ward (2003) argues that teams exist to get a job done. Meeting the needs of patients requires nurses to take account of not only the roles of the members of their immediate team but also those of the extended interprofessional team, other teams and agencies and, importantly, the needs of the patients (Elliott and Koubel, 2009).

Lewin's (1947) model of change is often cited in management training. It is a simple model that reflects many of the aspects of change that need to be accounted for if change is to be managed successfully.

Lewin's model is called 'the freeze, unfreeze, freeze model', and is perhaps best thought of by thinking about a block of ice. If you want to change a block of ice from a cube shape to a sphere, then the best way to change it is to first unfreeze it, and then (while it is liquid) pour it into a new mould before freezing it again. Similarly, if you want to instigate change in people, you must find a way to get them from where they are now (the initial freeze stage) to where you want them to be by getting them to 'unfreeze' the way they think and behave, to adapt to a new perspective, and then freeze again in the new way of behaving or thinking.

What, then, does this tell us about how to get evidence-based changes adopted by the teams or organisations in which we work? First, there is the issue of identifying what we do now and why (the initial freeze). This allows us to explore the quality of what we do. In order to change, we need to decide what it is we want to change, why and how.

This first stage is all about communication and setting the vision for how things might be and what outcomes we might expect if we decide to change. One example might be the introduction of a new pressure ulcer dressing in the general ward. First of all, we might undertake an audit of the use of such dressings now. This audit might include quantifying how many dressings we use, how much each dressing costs, how frequently the dressing has to be changed, how easy the dressing is to use, the effectiveness of the dressing (how long a particular grade of ulcer takes to heal), the acceptability of the dressing to the patient, the incidence of infection in patients using the dressing and any associated costs of cleansing the wound. This information provides benchmarking data against which we might trial a new dressing.

We may then decide that we want to speed up the process of healing or reduce the incidence of infection-related complications in patients with similar ulcers. A review of the literature on pressure ulcers and discussions with experienced and expert staff in wound management might then be used to understand the options available. Some understanding of the pros and cons of the new approach and some ideas about exactly what it is that we want to achieve will create the vision for how things might be. During this stage it is important to engage all the team in the process so they know what the purpose of the change is and can contribute ideas and insights as well as discuss fears and potential barriers.

During the initial planning stage strategies such as education (Haynes and Haines, 1998), clinical supervision and team meetings might be helpful in overcoming resistance. These strategies also promote inclusivity and demonstrate a commitment to being 'other regarding' as well as exploiting the potential benefits of working with others.

The process of trialling the change – again, collecting data on the variables identified earlier – is the 'unfreezing' stage. 'Unfreezing' is about trying the alternatives and exploring what advantages might be gained and what problems might arise. Again, it is important to include all the team, as they will then be able to contribute to the evaluation of the change. Failure to include the team can create mistrust and fear; it may lead to some people doing things in a different way from everyone else and can derail the whole process.

As ever, the role of the patient in this process is very important. We cannot know how comfortable the dressing is when in place or how much discomfort is associated with changing it unless we ask. Not only does this allow us to assess another one of our criteria for adopting the change, it again demonstrates a willingness to be 'other regarding' as identified in the dispositions of the evidence-based nurse in Chapter 1.

The move to consolidating practice (the second 'freeze') can then occur when the change has been assessed. It is worthy of note that not all potential evidence-based

Table 8.3: Managing the process of changing the choice of dressing

Define the need	Quantify use, cost, frequency of changes needed, healing times, incidence of infection. Establish ease of use and patient preference.
Plan ahead	Review the literature. Consult the experts. Define what a good outcome might look like.
Involve the team	Use team meetings. Consider clinical supervision. Use the expertise in the team. Provide education and training.
Trial the new product	Involve all the team. Get feedback on ease of use and patient preference and tolerability.
Assess the feedback	Decide as a team if the change is worth making.
Evaluate practice	Make the change or stick with what you have: evaluate the feeling of the team and move towards establishing the new or re-establishing the old practice.

changes to practice can, or are, adopted in practice because of local issues, such as expertise, cost or user preference (Gomm, 2002a, 2000b).

For the evidence-based nurse there is little to be gained from going it alone with a change in practice. The benefits that might accrue from advancing and developing practice can only be fully realised if they are adopted by the whole team (see Table 8.3).

Benefits to the patient

It seems only right to end this book with some thoughts about how evidence-based practice can benefit patients. Throughout the book we have seen that evidence is not merely about the blind adoption of changes to practice identified from within research papers. We have seen that our own experience, the shared experiences of others and research serve as sources of evidence, and that working with others, reflection, the ability to critique research and a conscientious clinical decision-making process help us to process information into something that informs care. We have also noted at various points along the way that the purpose of adopting an evidential approach to nursing care is not merely about ticking academic or regulatory boxes. It is about benefiting our patients.

What is clear from the ideas contained within this book is that the evidence-based nurse who takes account of the dispositions and influences on practice identified in the model in Chapter 1 will operate in a way that benefits patients in two important ways.

The first is by including them in the process of generating the evidence base – that is to say, taking account of their experience and knowledge. As well as paying attention to the patient's experience, the evidence-based nurse will also be patient-centred in the decision-making process, taking account of patient preference and perceived need as well as other forms of knowledge.

The second benefit to the patient is perhaps more obvious in that evidence-based nursing care is good-quality care – it is care that is grounded in carefully generated knowledge. High-quality, acceptable, patient-centred care is, after all, what we should all be aiming for.

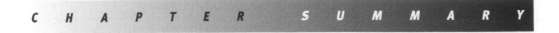

C H A P T E R   S U M M A R Y

The process of getting evidence into practice is one of change. Reasons for adopting evidence in practice include improving what we do and how we do it. There are also good moral and ethical imperatives for this.

In this chapter we have explored some of the strategies we can use individually and collectively to implement change in the clinical setting. The fundamental purpose for the identification and adoption of evidence is quite simply the improvement of practice.

Throughout the book we have presented a series of challenges to becoming evidence-based, and identified a number of strategies and an overall framework that will support the development of this.

Activities: brief outline answers

Activity 8.2: Critical thinking (page 119)

The activity of nursing is unique because of what it does and the people who do it. What nurses do is wide and varied, and tends to be whatever needs to be done. This ability to see the big picture and act upon it (being holistic) and to know where to go to get help to achieve this goal is what sets nursing apart. Few other professions can truly claim to stand with the patient at the heart of care, displaying humanity and humility while simultaneously interacting with other professions to achieve good care outcomes. The potential for achieving this uniqueness relies heavily on the dispositions and abilities of the individual nurse. It is a potential that becoming evidential, in the broad sense that we have demonstrated in this book, can allow us to achieve.

Activity 8.3: Reflection (page 120)

Many nurses do not like change because they understand the practices that they are used to and they can predict the likely outcomes of the activities with which they are engaged. Change takes energy, and when people are already working hard the energy that is needed to undertake change is alarming, especially when the benefits of the change are not thought to include reducing the time and effort that people have to put into their work.

Activity 8.5: Critical thinking (page 122)

Failure to adopt an evidential approach to nursing practice will lead to a number of detrimental consequences, some of which are listed here:

- nurse acting under the authority of others rather than autonomously;
- a poor public perception of nursing;
- job dissatisfaction;
- poor use of resources;
- poor outcomes for patients;
- inability to justify what we do and how we do it;
- inability to meet the governance agenda in hospitals.

Activity 8.6: Reflection (page 124)

It is likely that the perceptions of many of us about the people who care for us are based on the impressions we form of them as individuals. This perception will be formed on the basis of their appearance, how they talk to us and who they are. As with all healthcare professionals, the public perception of who they are is based not only on face-to-face meetings but also on their portrayal in the media. This media image is, at least in part, driven by the scandals and other negative events that occur. There are numerous examples where the competence of nursing staff to deliver care and recognise abuse and standards of personal and professional conduct have made the headlines; these most certainly impact on the image of the profession as a whole. There is little doubt that some of these issues of competence and behaviour are linked to the lack of commitment of some individuals to providing high-quality evidence-informed care.

Activity 8.7: Critical thinking (page 126)

Reasons why nursing needs to adapt to change include the constantly changing environments of care, which include: the emergence of new diseases and treatments for diseases; the changing demographics within society; changing expectations within society; and increasing professionalisation of nursing through extended and specialist roles.

Activity 8.8: Reflection (page 127)

There are many simple personal strategies that can improve your ability to function as an evidence-based nurse. These strategies include identifying simple sources of evidence you can use to inform your practice. You might, for example, set up e-mail alerts from some of the many nursing and medical websites that provide updates of the most recent articles and research in the area in which you work; you might subscribe to a nursing journal; better still, you might start or join a journal club. Clinical supervision is a powerful tool for self-development, as is engaging in focused conversations about care with your clinical mentor. Service users (patients) provide a great source of insight into how care is experienced and what it is like to be ill. Perhaps you might keep a reflective diary that allows you not only to put on paper what you are thinking and feeling but to focus on developing the above strategies to enhance your practice.

Activity 8.9: Critical thinking (page 128)

Critical thinking often arises out of repeated exposure to things. This exposure allows us to start to see connections between issues as well as to explore our thinking and feelings. The theory–practice gap can be a devastating realisation for novice nurses who see it as immoral and illogical. Experience and education enable us to reflect on some of the reasons for it, which include many of the barriers to change we have already identified. This process of realisation speeds up as we start to form theories and understanding of reality and start to see the bigger picture and where things fit into this bigger picture. Applying ourselves to thinking about and understanding our realities is critical thinking; it helps us identify why things occur and place them in a greater scheme of understanding and realisation.

Knowledge review

Now that you have completed the chapter, how would you rate your knowledge of the following topics?

	Good	Adequate	Poor
1. The reasons why adopting evidence-based practice for nursing care is important.			
2. The barriers to adopting evidence.			
3. The steps that may need to be taken to get evidence into practice.			
4. Why it is important for you to adopt evidence-based nursing.			

Where you're not confident in your knowledge of a topic, what will you do next?

Further reading

Gomm, R and Davies, C (eds) (2000) *Using evidence in health and social care*. London: Sage.
An easy-to-read overview of many of the topics raised in this book.

Koubel, G and Bungay, H (eds) (2009) *The challenge of person-centred care: an interprofessional perspective*. Basingstoke: Palgrave.
One of the few books that considers patient-centred care in the interprofessional context.

National Institute for Health and Clinical Excellence (NICE) (2007) *How to change practice: Understand, identify and overcome barriers to change*. London: NICE.
This document is simply laid out and easy to read, and can be accessed through the NICE website (see below) by typing the title and first word of the subtitle into the search box on the top right.

Price, B and Harrington, A (2010) *Critical thinking and writing for nursing students*. Exeter: Learning Matters.
A book for student nurses on how to think critically.

Useful websites

www.businessballs.com/changemanagement.htm A management theory website with some accessible ideas on change management.
www.nice.org.uk The website of the National Institute for Health and Clinical Excellence.

A generic research critiquing framework with additional paradigm specific questions

The first section of this framework can be applied to all research. The following sections apply specifically to qualitative and quantitative research, and apply questions in a manner specific to these methodologies.

Questions that apply to all research

Background issues

Title
Does this identify:

- the type of people to whom the research is being applied?
- the research question or aims?
- the methodology or data-collection method?
- the main finding(s) of the study?

Author credentials
Can you identify the author's:

- qualifications?
- professional background?
- current job?
- experience of doing similar research?

Core research issues

The question
- Does the introduction and background to the study identify the need for the research to be done?
- Can you identify the purpose of the research (its aim, objective, question or hypothesis)?

Methodology, methods and sampling
- Given the question, does the research paradigm and methodology chosen make sense?

- Even if 'yes', are there alternative methodologies that might be appropriate as well?
- Given the methodology identified (if any), do the research data-collection methods fit?
- Even if 'yes', are there alternative methods that might be appropriate as well?
- With regard to the sample:
    - Is the method of recruiting reasonable?
    - Is the sample of the right size?
    - Does the sample represent the people the study is about?
    - Even if 'yes', are there alternative strategies that might have made the process as good or better?

Results, conclusions and discussion

- Is the approach to analysis of results consistent with the type of data collected?
- With regard to the results:
    - Is it apparent how the data were analysed?
    - Are these clear?
    - Do they reflect what the researchers set out to answer?
- Does the discussion:
    - reflect the results?
    - reflect the purpose of the research?
    - identify practical issues that have impaired the research?
    - identify compromises that have been made to allow the research to proceed?
    - only make claims about things the research set out to answer?
    - explain why the results have occurred?
    - contain additional results?
- Does the conclusion:
    - only discuss what the aim(s) of the research were about?
    - reflect the results and discussion?
    - identify and compare the results to other similar research?
    - identify and compare the results to existing and potential policy?
    - suggest possibilities for future research?

Ethical issues

- Have the researchers:
    - demonstrated the research is necessary?
    - gained ethics approval?
    - demonstrated concern for confidentiality and anonymity?
    - shown concern for informed consent including:
        - freedom from coercion (or appearance of potential coercion);
        - information giving;
        - freedom of choice;
        - right of participants to withdraw;
        - extra concern for potentially vulnerable participants?
- Have the researchers shown concern for the ethical principles of:
    - doing good?
    - avoiding unnecessary harm?
    - respecting participant autonomy (see also consent)?
    - respect for fairness?

Additional questions that apply to qualitative research

When critiquing qualitative research, these additional questions, using terms specific to qualitative research, *must* also be considered.

Rigour

- Has the research process has been fully explained in a transparent manner that is clear from the article?

Dependability

- Has the study been undertaken in a consistent manner?
  - Have all researchers used the same procedures?

Credibility

- Have the researchers checked the level of agreement with their findings?
  - Did the researchers check their interpretation with the participants and/or other professionals?

Confirmability

- Has the data been dealt with in a neutral manner?

Transferability

- Does other research appear to support the findings?
  - If no, are the reasons for the difference explained coherently?

Additional questions that apply to quantitative research

When critiquing quantitative research, these additional questions, using terms specific to quantitative research, *must* also be considered.

Bias

- Have the researchers identified and dealt with potential bias within the study design and execution? Specific biases may include:
  - behavioural bias;
  - measurement bias;
  - recall bias;
  - response bias;
  - **sampling bias**;
  - selection bias.

Confounding

- Are there alternative explanations for what has occurred in the study?

Validity

- Does the study measure what it says it will measure and do the data-collection tools do what they say they do?

Reliability

- Have the researchers demonstrated that the data collection has occurred in a consistent and reproducible manner?

Generalisability and representativeness

- Where the researchers have claimed the study is generalisable, is the study sample representative of the people they claim the findings apply to?

Glossary

anonymity: the process of protecting or hiding an individual's true identity.

autonomy: the freedom, and in some senses the ability, to choose what we will do with our lives and our bodies. It implies freedom from pressure from others.

behavioural bias: bias that occurs when people within a study behave in a given manner because of some underlying reason that usually affects all similar individuals.

beneficence: the ethical principle of doing good.

benign: non-cancerous.

bias: in the context of research, anything in the design or undertaking of a study that causes an untruth to occur in the study, potentially affecting the outcome of the study.

biographic research: research based on the accounts of individuals who have experienced a particular life event, recounted primarily in their own words.

biopsy: removal of a small sample of tissue.

capacity: relates to the ability of an individual to understand information given in the consent process.

case study: a study that explores individual or small, similar accounts of a phenomenon or disease and may be either quantitative or qualitative.

cathartic interventions: verbal and non-verbal skills enabling others to express feelings.

clinical governance: a system of audit and other checks health services use to check on and improve their services.

cognitively: refers to the ability to be able to think rationally and provide meaning.

confidentiality: only divulging information that has been given by a patient to the people that the patient has agreed that the information may be shared with, and not sharing the information beyond this group. It is a cornerstone of nursing practice.

confirmability: the degree to which the results of a qualitative enquiry can be confirmed by others.

confounding: occurs when alternative explanations for an outcome in a study are not accounted for. Confounding variables are always independently associated with both the exposure and the outcome being measured. For example, an increased risk of cancer of the pancreas is associated with both smoking and coffee drinking, and smokers tend to drink more coffee than non-smokers.

consent: the process of allowing people to make choices about what they do and what is done to them when they have a full understanding of the facts and are free from external pressures.

convenience sample: a sample taken from a set of individuals who are easily accessed.

credible/credibility: believable; a term used in qualitative research to suggest that the research undertaken actually answers what it set out to answer because of the quality of the way in which the research has been done.

cross-sectional studies: studies that take place within a defined period of time and are used to determine the prevalence of disease or an exposure to a disease.

data saturation: the point during the qualitative research process at which no more new data (ideas, concepts or themes) are emerging. It is at this point that the researcher is most confident that they have collected all the data they can within their sample.

deductive: refers to research that sets out to prove an existing idea or hypothesis – to explore the truthfulness of the original idea.

dependability: consistency in the data collection, if more than one researcher – or data-collection method – is used.

dependent variable: the outcome variable of the study, which occurs as a result of the independent variable having occurred.

descriptive statistics: the use of statistics to describe the frequencies and pattern of numbers with a data set.

embedded knowledge: practice knowledge that is rooted in clinical contexts as they continually adjust to new challenges in addressing healthcare needs.

embodied knowledge: personal knowledge that is rooted in a person's individual identity as they continually interact with others in performing healthcare roles.

empirical: the notion of discovering new things using the senses or, in the case of research, different methods.

essence: the nature of something.

ethnography: a qualitative research methodology concerned with how people interact in groups.

exploratory qualitative study: a study that uses qualitative methods, but does not identify a specific qualitative methodology – often called a generic qualitative study.

generalise/generalisability/generalisable/generalised: refers to the ability of the findings of a study to be extrapolated to the wider population.

generic qualitative study: a study that uses qualitative methods, but does not identify a specific qualitative methodology – often called an exploratory study.

gestalt: moment of insight and understanding.

grounded theory: a qualitative, inductive research approach used to generate theories in the area of human interactions.

Hawthorne effect: occurs when people respond in the manner in which they believe they should when confronted by a researcher asking questions. The Hawthorne effect can bias a study.

homogeneous/homogeneity: the same – as in homogenized milk, which is the same consistency throughout: there is no cream at the top.

hypothesis: an idea that quantitative research sets out to prove.

independent variable: the causal variable in a study, which may be manipulated during a study.

inductive: refers to the process of developing a theory or hypothesis by first collecting and examining the evidence and seeing where this leads.

inferential statistics: statistics that are used to draw conclusions about the level of association between two or more variables within a study.

informative interventions: communicating skills enabling others to exercise informed choice.

justice: acting fairly so that people are treated generally in the same way.

longitudinal: taking place over a period of time.

mammogram: X-ray of the breast.

mean: also called the average; the sum of all the observations in a data set divided by the number of observations.

measurement bias: occurs when something is measured incorrectly in a consistent manner.

median: the middle value of an ordered set of observations.

methodologies/methodology: the broad approaches to research that provide the general framework of the enquiry.

methods: in the sense they are used in this book, the specific tools used to collect data during the research process, e.g. a questionnaire.

non-maleficence: the ethical principle of avoiding doing harm, perhaps better thought of as 'first do no harm'.

null hypothesis: the opposite of what the researcher actually expects to find. It is stated in this way in order to aid statistical analysis and to help demonstrate management of potential bias.

paradigm: in the sense that the term is applied in this book, the philosophical position that is taken within the research.

phenomenological: lived experience from which phenomena may be deduced.

phenomenology: a research methodology within qualitative research concerned with understanding the 'essence' of an experience or perceived reality from the point of view of someone experiencing the phenomenon of interest.

probability sampling: the selection of people from a large potential study population that allows everyone the same chance of being included in the study.

prospective: going forward in time.

pulse oximetry: measurement of oxygen saturation of haemoglobin in red blood cells.

purposive sampling/purposively: refers to a method of sampling within qualitative research whereby people are chosen for inclusion because they meet the *purpose* of the study. This means they have experience of the phenomenon being studied.

qualitative paradigm: a paradigm associated with the social and psychological sciences and interested in discovering truths about how people experience the world and why.

qualitative research: research that explores attitudes, opinions, experiences or behaviours through interviews, focus groups or observation.

quantitative paradigm: a paradigm that views the world in a conventionally scientific sense and that is interested in proving associations, correlations and cause and effect.

quantitative research: research that seeks to discover relationships between variables in a statistical way.

randomised controlled trial (RCT): a specific form of experiment that is used in the clinical setting in order to compare the usefulness of two or more interventions.

recall bias: occurs when individuals in a study have to rely on their memory in order to answer certain questions. Such biases are created when people who are ill, or have another reason to remember an exposure, are better at recalling events than people who are not. Last (1995) gives the example of mothers of children with leukaemia being better at recalling having had X-rays while pregnant than mothers of children who are not.

reflection-in-action: thinking and learning while actively engaged in an activity (thinking on your feet).

reflection-on-action: thinking through and reflecting on an activity after the event.

reflexive/reflexivity: the conscious engagement on the part of the researcher in being open to and expressing their own biases and opinions that might affect the carrying out and interpretation of the research.

reliability/reliable: refers to whether a method of data collection, or measurement, will repeatedly give the same results if used by the same person more than once or by two or more people when measuring the same phenomenon.

representative: in sampling means the people included in the study are broadly similar to the population (or group) that the sample is taken from.

response bias: occurs when individuals respond to a question within a study in a particular way because they think that the answer they are giving is what the researcher wants to hear.

retrospective: looking back in time.

rigour/rigorous: a term used in qualitative research that suggests that the research process has been undertaken in a well-thought-through, explained and transparent manner.

sampling bias: occurs when the selection of a sample for a study may exclude certain groups of people in a systematic manner; for example, an online survey will exclude all those people who do not have internet access.

saturation: see data saturation.

selection bias: bias can happen as a result of an action occurring on one side of a study and not the other. If researchers were allowed to decide which participants had which intervention in a study, it is possible that they might select patients they thought would do better in the study or try harder to follow a regime; this would be called selection bias.

study population: all people who fit the study inclusion/exclusion criteria.

study sample: the people who are eventually chosen for the study.

supportive interventions: verbal and non-verbal skills enabling others to feel respected.

theoretical sampling: occurs as the researcher builds new theories and ideas from the data they have collected and test this theory by interviewing more subjects to see if the new theory still holds true. Usually only a feature of grounded theory research. Also called 'handy sampling'.

tracheal stricture: narrowing of the trachea.

tracheostomy tube: a tube inserted into the trachea to aid breathing.

transferable: refers to how well the findings of a qualitative study might transfer to other, similar cases. This is generally regarded as having less power than generalisability.

triangulation: a technique used to increase the credibility of research by using research approaches from both research paradigms, or more than one data-collection method. It helps demonstrate the accuracy of what is found in much the same way that providing a longitude and latitude reading helps pinpoint a location on a map.

validity/valid: refers to the ability of a method (or data-collection technique) to measure what it is supposed to be measuring. For example, we know that a thermometer (if placed correctly for long enough) will measure temperature, but it is not easy to be certain that a questionnaire designed to measure quality of life actually does so because it is not always easy to define what quality of life actually is.

variable: literally something that varies, such as eye colour or age. In the research sense it refers to the thing being explored within the study. See also **dependent variable** and **independent variable**.

vegetative state: a persistent coma.

verbatim: word for word, literally as something was said.

vital signs: measurement of consciousness, temperature, respiration, pulse and blood pressure.

References

Baines, L (1998) Listening to the evidence. *Nursing Standard*, 12 (23): 20.

Barber, C, McLaughlin, N, and Wood, J (2009) Self-awareness: the key to person-centred care? in Koubel, G and Bungay, H (eds) *The challenge of person-centred care: an interprofessional perspective*. Basingstoke: Palgrave.

Barker, J (2010) *Evidence-based practice for nurses*. Los Angeles CA: Sage Publications.

Barnett, R (2000) *Realizing the university in an age of supercomplexity*. Milton Keynes: Society for Research into Higher Education and Open University Press.

Beauchamp, TL and Childress, JF (2007) *Principles of Biomedical Ethics* (6th ed.). Oxford: Oxford University Press.

Benjamin, M and Curtis, J (1992) *Ethics in nursing* (3rd ed.). New York: Oxford University Press.

Benner, P (1984) *From novice to expert: excellence and power in clinical nursing practice*. Menlo Park CA: Addison-Wesley Publishing Company.

Berwick, DM (2003) Disseminating innovations in health care. *The Journal of the American Medical Association*, 289 (15): 1969–75.

Bloomfield, J, Roberts, J, and While, A (2010) The effect of computer-assisted learning versus conventional teaching methods on the acquisition and retention of handwashing theory and skills in pre-qualification nursing students: a randomised controlled trial. *International Journal of Nursing Studies*, 47: 287–94.

Bolton, G (2010) *Reflective practice: writing and professional development* (3rd ed.). Los Angeles CA: Sage.

Braden, R, Reichow, S and Halm, MA (2009) The use of the essential oil Lavandin to reduce preoperative anxiety in surgical patients. *Journal of PeriAnesthesia Nursing*, 24 (6): 348–55.

Brechin, A (2000) Introducing critical practice, in Brechin, A, Brown, H and Eby, MA (eds) *Critical practice in health and social care*. London: Sage.

Brookfield, S (2005) *The power of critical theory for adult learning and teaching*. Milton Keynes: Open University Press

Brown, GD (1995) Understanding barriers to basing nursing practice upon research: a communication model approach. *Journal of Advanced Nursing*, 21: 154–7.

Buswell, C (1998) Feeling is believing. *Nursing Standard*, 12 (23): 20.

Cangelosi, PR (2008) Learning portfolios: giving meaning to practice. *Nurse Educator*, 33 (3): 125–7.

Care Quality Commission (2009) *Review of the involvement and action taken by health bodies in relation to the case of Baby P*. London: CQC.

Carel, H (2008) *Illness*. Stocksfield: Acumen.

Carper, BA (1978) Fundamental patterns of knowing in nursing. *Advances in Nursing Science*, 1 (1): 13–23.

Centre for Change and Innovation (2003) *Talking matters: developing the communication skills of doctors*. Edinburgh: Scottish Executive.

Connelly, N and Seden, J (2003) What service users say about services: the implications for managers, in Henderson, J and Atkinson, D (eds) *Managing Care in Context*. London: Routledge.

Couchman, W and Dawson, J (1995) *Nursing and healthcare research: a practical guide* (2nd ed.). London: Scutari Press.

Coughlan, M, Cronin, P and Ryan, F (2007) Step-by-step guide to critiquing research: part 1: quantitative research. *British Journal of Nursing*, 16 (11): 658–63.

Craig, JV and Smyth, RL (eds) (2002) *The evidence-based manual for nurses*. Edinburgh: Churchill Livingstone.

Delanty, G and Strydom, P (eds.) (2003) *Philosophies of social science: the classic and contemporary readings*. Maidenhead: Open University Press.

DH (Department of Health) (1989) *Working for patients*. London: HMSO.

DH (1991) *The patient's charter*. London: HMSO.

DH (2000) *The NHS plan: A plan for investment, a plan for reform*. London: Her Majesty's Stationery Office (HMSO).

DH (2001) *The NHS Plan*. London: HMSO.

DH (2007) *Privacy and dignity: a report by the Chief Nursing Officer into mixed sex accommodation in hospitals*. London: DH.

Dubler, NN (1992) Individual advocacy as a governing principle. *Journal of Case Management*, 13: 82–6.

Dworkin, R (1993) *Life's dominion: an argument about abortion and euthanasia*. London: HarperCollins.

Elliott, P (2009) *Infection control: a psychosocial approach to changing practice*. Oxford: Radcliffe Publishing.

Elliott, P and Koubel, G (2009) What is person-centred care? in Koubel, G and Bungay, H (eds) *The challenge of person-centred care: an interprofessional perspective*. Basingstoke: Palgrave, pp29–50.

Ellis, P (1996) Exploring the concept of acting in the patient's best interests. *British Journal of Nursing*, 5 (17): 1072–4.

Ellis, P (2010) *Understanding research for nursing students*. Exeter: Learning Matters.

Fasnacht, PH (2003) Creativity: a refinement of the concept for nursing practice. *Journal of Advanced Nursing*, 41 (2): 195–202.

Flanagan, OJ (1981) Psychology, progress, and the problem of reflexivity: a study in the epistemological foundations of psychology. *Journal of the History of the Behavioral Sciences*, 17: 375–86.

Gadamer, HG (1989) *Truth and method* (2nd ed.). London: Sheed and Ward.

Gawande, A. (2009) *The checklist manifesto: how to get things right*. New York: Metropolitan Books.

George, SR and Thomas, SP (2010) Lived experience of diabetes among older, rural people. *Journal of Advanced Nursing*, 66 (5), 1092–100.

Gerish, K and Lacey, A (2006) *The research process in nursing* (5th ed.). Oxford: Blackwell.

Glaser, BG and Strauss, AL (1967) *The discovery of grounded theory: strategies for qualitative research*. Chicago IL: Aldine Publishing Company.

Gomm, R (2000a) Would it work here? in Gomm, R and Davies, C (eds) *Using evidence in health and social care*. London: Sage.

Gomm, R (2000b) Should we afford it? in Gomm, R and Davies, C (eds) *Using evidence in health and social care*. London: Sage.

González, J. and Wagenaar, R. (2003) *Tuning educational structures in Europe: final report pilot project – Phase 1*. Bilbao: University of Deusto.

Greenhalgh, T (2006) *How to read a paper: the basics of evidence-based medicine* (3rd ed.). Oxford: Blackwell.

Haynes, B and Haines, A (1998) Barriers and bridges to evidence-based clinical practice. *British Medical Journal*, 317 (7153): 273–6.

Hayward, J (1979) *Information: a prescription against pain*. London: Royal College of Nursing.

Health and Safety Executive (1974) *The Health and Safety at Work Act 1974*. London: HSE. Available online at: www.hse.gov.uk/legislation/hswa.htm (accessed 27 May 2010).

Healthcare Commission (2007) *Investigation into outbreaks of Clostridium difficile at Maidstone and Tunbridge Wells NHS Trust*. London: Commission for Healthcare Audit and Inspection.

Hek, G and Moule, P (2006) *Making sense of research: an introduction for health and social care practitioners*. London: Sage.

Heron, J. (1989) *Six category intervention analysis* (3rd ed.). Guildford: Human Potential Resource Group – University of Surrey.

Heron, J (1996) *Co-operative inquiry: research into the human condition*. London: Sage Publications.

Hilton, S, Bedford, H, Calnan, M and Hunt, K (2009) Competency, confidence and conflicting evidence: key issues affecting health visitors' use of research evidence in practice, *BMC Nursing*, 8 (4) doi: 10.1186/1472–6955-8-4.

Holmes, TH and Rahe, RH (1967) The social readjustments rating scales. *Journal of Psychosomatic Research*, 11: 213–18.

Hopson, B and Adams, J (1976) *Transition: understanding and managing personal change*. London, Martin Robertson.

Janesick, VJ (2003) *The choreography of qualitative research design*, in Denzin, NK and Lincoln, YS (eds) *Strategies of qualitative inquiry* (2nd ed.). Thousand Oaks CA: Sage Publications, pp 46–79.

Jansson, W, Nordberg, G, and Grafstrom, M (2001) Patterns of elderly spousal caregiving in dementia care: an observational study. *Journal of Advanced Nursing*, 34 (6): 804–12.

Jarvis, P (2006) *Towards a comprehensive theory of human learning: lifelong learning and the learning society, volume 1*. London: Routledge.

Jasper, M (2003) *Foundations in nursing and health care: beginning reflective practice*. Cheltenham: Nelson Thornes.

Johnson, JL and Ratner, PA (1997) The nature of knowledge used in nursing practice, in Thorne, SE and Hayes, VE (eds) *Nursing praxis: knowledge and action*. London: Sage.

Jolley, J (2010) *Introducing research and evidence-based practice for nurses*. London: Pearson.

Jones, AM (2003) Changes in practice at the nurse–doctor interface: using focus groups to explore the perceptions of first level nurses working in an acute care setting. *Journal of Clinical Nursing*, 12: 124–31.

Kemmis, S and McTaggert, R (2003) Participatory action research, in Denzin, NK and Lincoln, YS (eds) *Strategies of qualitative enquiry* (2nd ed.). Thousand Oaks CA: Sage Publications, pp 336–96.

Kilian, C, Salmoni, A, Ward-Griffin, C, and Kloseck, M (2008) Perceiving falls within a family context: a focused ethnographic approach. *Canadian Journal on Aging*, 27 (4): 331–45.

Kitson, A, Ahmed, LB, Harvey, G, Seers, K and Thompson, DR (1996) From research to practice: one organisational model for promoting research-based practice. *Journal of Advanced Nursing*, 23: 430–40.

Kitson, A, Harvey, G and McCormack, B (1998) Enabling the implementation of evidence-based practice: a conceptual framework. *Quality in Health Care*, 7: 149–58.

Last, JM (1995) *A dictionary of epidemiology* (3rd ed.). Oxford: Oxford University Press.

L'Eplattenier, N (2001) Tracing the development of critical thinking in baccalaureate nursing students. *Journal of the New York State Nurses Association*, 32 (2): 27–32.

Lewin, K (1947) Frontiers in group dynamics: concept, method, and reality in social science. *Human Relations*, 1: 5–42.

Lobiondo-Wood, G and Haber, J (1998) *Nursing research: methods, critical appraisal, and utilization* (4th ed.). St Louis MO: Mosby.

Macnee, CL and McCabe, S (2008) *Understanding nursing research: reading and using research in evidence-based practice* (2nd ed.). London: Wolters Kluwer/Lippincott, Williams and Wilkins.

Maguire, P and Pitceathly, C (2002) Key communication skills and how to acquire them. *British Medical Journal*, 325: 697–700.

Manias, E and Street, A (2000) Legitimation of nurses' knowledge through policies and protocols in clinical practice. *Journal of Advanced Nursing*, 32 (6):1467–75.

McKibbon, KA (1998) Evidence-based practice. *Bulletin of the Medical Library Association*, 86 (3): 396–401.

McNiff, J and Whitehead, J (2002) *Action research: principles and practice* (2nd ed.). London: Routledge/Falmer.

Meads, G, Barr, H, Scott, R, Ashcroft, J, and Wild, A (2005) *The case for inter-professional collaboration*. Oxford: Blackwell.

Meadus, RJ (2007) Adolescents coping with mood disorder: a grounded theory study. *Journal of Psychiatric and Mental Health Nursing*, 14: 209–17.

Merrill, B and West, L (2009) *Using biographical methods in social research*. Los Angeles: Sage Publications.

Milton, CL (2007) Evidence-based practice: ethical questions for nursing. *Nursing Science Quarterly*, 20 (2): 123–6.

Muir, N (2004) Clinical decision-making: theory and practice. *Nursing Standard*, 18 (36): 47–52.

NICE (National Institute for Health and Clinical Excellence) (2007) *How to change practice: Understand, identify and overcome barriers to change*. London: NICE.

Nilsson Kajermo, K, Nordstrom, G, Krusebrant, A, and Bjorvell, H (1998) Barriers to and facilitators of research utilization, as perceived by a group of registered nurses in Sweden. *Journal of Advanced Nursing*, 27: 798–807.

NMC (Nursing and Midwifery Council) (2004) Standards of proficiency for pre-registration nursing education. London: NMC.

NMC (2008) *The Code: Standards of conduct, performance and ethics for nurses and midwives*. London: NMC.

NMC (2009a) *Guidance on professional conduct for nursing and midwifery students*. London: NMC.

NMC (2009b) *Record keeping: guidance for nurses and midwives*. London: NMC.

NMC (Nursing and Midwifery Council) (2010) *Standards for pre-registration nursing education*. London: NMC.

Nolan, D and Ellis, P (2008) Communication and advocacy, in Howatson-Jones, L and Ellis, P (eds) *Outpatient, day surgery and ambulatory care*. Chichester: Wiley-Blackwell.

OPSI (Office of Public Sector Information) (1989) *The Children Act, 1989*. London: OPSI. Available online at: www.opsi.gov.uk/acts/acts1989/ukpga_19890041_en_1 (accessed: 27 May 2010).

OPSI (1998) *The Data Protection Act, 1998*. London: OPSI. Available online at: www.opsi.gov.uk/acts/acts1998/ukpga_19980029_en_1 (accessed 27 May 2010).

Øvretveit, J, Mathias, P and Thompson, T (1997) *Interprofessional working for health and social care*. Basingstoke: MacMillan.

Oxford English Dictionaries (1996) *The Oxford Concise English Dictionary*. Oxford: Oxford University Press.

Parahoo, K (2006) *Nursing research: principles, process and issues* (2nd ed.). London: Palgrave Macmillan.

Parsons, L and Stanley, M (2008) The lived experience of occupational adaptation following acquired brain injury for people living in a rural area. *Australian Occupational Therapy Journal*, 55 (4): 231–8.

Patients Association (2009) *Patients not numbers, people not statistics*. [on-line] Available online at: www.patients-association.org.uk/DBIMGS/file/Patients%20not%20numbers,%20people%20not%20statistics.pdf (accessed 26 October 2009).

Pattison, S (2001) Health and healing in an age of science, in Seale, C, Pattison, S and Davey, B, *Medical knowledge, doubt and certainty*. Buckingham: Open University Press, pp14–42.

Petticrew, M and Roberts, H (2003) Evidence, hierarchies and typologies: horses for courses. *Journal of Epidemiology and Community Health*, 57 (7): 527–9.

Polit, DF and Beck, CT (2006) *Essentials of nursing research: methods, appraisal and utilization* (6th ed.). London: Lippincott, Williams and Wilkins.

Polit, DF and Beck, CT (2008) *Nursing research: generating and accessing evidence for nursing practice* (8th ed.). London: Lippincott, Williams and Wilkins.

Pronovost, P, Needham, D, Berenholtz, S et al. (2006) An intervention to reduce catheter-related bloodstream infections in the ICU. *New England Journal of Medicine*, 355: 2725–32.

Robson, V, Dodd, S and Thomas, S (2009) Standardized antibacterial honey (Medihoney™) with standard therapy in wound care: randomized clinical trial. *Journal of Advanced Nursing*, 65 (3): 565–75.

Rodgers, S (1994) An exploratory study of research utilization by nurses in general medical and surgical wards. *Journal of Advanced Nursing*, 20: 904–11.

Rogers, EM (1962) *Diffusion of Innovations*, Glencoe: Free Press.

Roose, GA and John, AM (2003) A focus group investigation into young children's understanding of mental health and their views on appropriate services for their age group. *Child Care, Health & Development*, 29 (6): 545–50.

Roper, N, Logan, WW and Tierney, AJ (2000) *The Roper-Logan-Tierney model of nursing: based on activities of living*. Edinburgh: Churchill Livingstone.

Rycroft-Malone, J, Seers, K, Titchen, A, Harvey, G, Kitson, A and McCormack, B (2004) An exploration of the factors that influence the implementation of evidence into practice. *Journal of Clinical Nursing*, 13: 913–24.

Sackett, DL, Rosenberg, WM, Gray, JA, Haynes, RB and Richardson, WS (1996) Evidence-based medicine: what it is and what it isn't. *British Medical Journal*, 312 (7023): 71–2.

Santrock, JW (2004) *Educational psychology* (2nd ed.), Saddle River NJ: Allyn and Bacon.

Scott, A (1998) Clinical governance relies on a change in culture. *British Journal of Nursing*, 7 (16): 940.

Sennett, R (2008) *The Craftsman*. London: Allen Lane/Penguin Books.

Sitzia, J, Cotterell, P and Richardson, A (2004) *Formative evaluation of the Cancer Partnership Project*. London: Macmillan Cancer Relief.

Standing, M (2005) Perceptions of clinical decision-making on a developmental journey from student to staff nurse. Unpublished PhD Thesis. Canterbury: University of Kent.

Standing, M (2007) Clinical decision-making skills on the developmental journey from student to registered nurse: a longitudinal inquiry. *Journal of Advanced Nursing* 60 (3): 257–69.

Standing, M (2010) Perceptions of clinical decision-making: a matrix model, in Standing, M (ed.) *Clinical judgement and decision-making: nursing and interprofessional healthcare.* Maidenhead: Open University Press.

Streubert Speziale, HJ and Carpenter, DR (2007) *Qualitative research in nursing: advancing the humanistic imperative,* (4th ed.). London: Lippincott, Williams and Wilkins.

Thompson, C, and Dowding, D (eds) (2002) *Clinical decision-making and judgement in nursing.* Edinburgh: Churchill Livingstone.

Thompson, C, McCaughan, D, Cullum, N, Sheldon, TA, Munhall, A and Thompson, DR (2001) Research information in nurses' clinical decision-making: What is useful? *Journal of Advanced Nursing,* 36 (3): 376–88.

Titchen, A, McGinley, M, and McCormack, B (2004) Blending self-knowledge and professional knowledge, in Higgs, J, Richardson, B and Abrandt Dahlgren, M. (eds) *Developing practice knowledge for health professionals.* Edinburgh: Butterworth Heinemann, pp. 107–26.

Ward, A (2003) Managing the team, in Seden, J and Reynolds, J, (eds) *Managing care in practice.* London: Routledge, pp33–56.

West, L, Alheit, P, Anderson, AS and Merrill, B (eds.) (2007) *Using biographical and life history approaches in the study of adult and lifelong learning: European perspectives.* Frankfurt am Main: Peter Lang.

Williams, G, Dean, P and Williams, E (2009) Do nurses really care? Confirming the stereotype with a case control study. *British Journal of Nursing,* 18 (3): 162–65.

Index